Pleasure People Diet

The
PLEASURE
PRINCIPLE
Diet

How to Lose Weight Permanently, Eating the Foods You Love

Robert E. Willner, M.D.

Prentice-Hall, Inc.   Englewood Cliffs, New Jersey

Prentice-Hall International, Inc., *London*
Prentice-Hall of Australia, Pty. Ltd., *Sydney*
Prentice-Hall Canada Inc., *Toronto*
Prentice-Hall of India Private Ltd., *New Delhi*
Prentice-Hall of Japan, Inc., *Tokyo*
Prentice-Hall of Southeast Asia Pte. Ltd., *Singapore*
Whitehall Books, Ltd., *Wellington, New Zealand*
Editora Prentice-Hall do Brasil, Ltda., *Rio de Janeiro*
Prentice-Hall Hispanoamericana, S. A., *Mexico*

© 1985 by
Robert E. Willner, M.D.

10   9   8   7   6   5

This book is a reference work based on research by the author.
The opinions expressed herein are not necessarily those of or en-
dorsed by the publisher. The directions stated in this book are in
no way to be considered as a substitute for consultation with a duly
licensed doctor.

Library of Congress Cataloging in Publication Data
Willner, Robert E.
  The pleasure principle diet.
  Includes index.
  1. Reducing diets. 2. Obesity. I. Title.
RM222.2.W456   1984   613.2'5   84-29121

ISBN 0-13-683442-6

ISBN 0-13-683434-5 {PBK}

Printed in the United States of America

To my wife Marcia, whose brilliant life was cruelly ended by brain cancer, and to our children, Bruce and Beth. They have added new meanings to love, new dimensions to life, and created infinite pleasure in both.

To all the gallant physicians and health professionals in preventive and alternative medicine who are leading the battle against the ultraconservatives in the medical establishment

No profit grows where is no pleasure *ta'en*
In brief, sir, study what you most affect.
William Shakespeare

Acknowledgments

How I wish that this page could be lit with neon lights and equipped with a sound system that would call the reader's attention to its existence and importance. Although it appears at the beginning of the book, it is written last. It is only after years of collecting material and doing research, followed by many months of writing, dictating, editing, rewriting, redictating, and reediting, that a writer can truly appreciate the many individuals who contribute to the final product. This book would have been impossible without the help and encouragement of my office manager, Lydia Gomes, and my office staff, Helen Shurgin, Mary DePathy, Beth Willner, and Camille Lombardo.

"Thanks" could never be enough to Al, "Dr. O" Olchak, my father-in-law and office controller, for his warm words of support and his deep friendship. He kept our office economically sound and solvent during the many months of writing. A special place of honor goes to a beautiful human being, Mrs. Anna Michaels, our incredible eighty-year-old housekeeper, adopted grandmother, and member of the family. Her "youth" has kept us all young, her hot drinks and snacks gave me energy during the long hours of work, and her beautiful Polish heritage formed the basis for the story in Act II, Scene 1, *Magic, Myths and Miracles.* I am indebted to Parkway General Hospital in North Miami Beach, Florida, for their cooperation in providing technical assistance, allowing me to use the services of Margaret Casey, hospital librarian, the hospital kitchen staff, and the staff of dietitians.

A manuscript must be reviewed many times in order to reflect soundness of concept, clarity of thought, and continuity of ideas and to create enjoyable reading. To be well-rounded, these reviews should be made by professionals and nonprofessionals. I deeply appreciate the constructive criticism given me through the efforts of the psychotherapists at the Douglas Gardens Out-Patient Mental Health Center in Miami, by Drs. Norman Reichenberg and Richard Greenbaum, both talented psychologists and very close friends, and by Diane Johnson, a patient who has probably read every diet book ever printed and has contributed invaluable comments from the layman's point of view.

Special thanks to Debbie Koenig for her constructive comments and proofreading.

A family physician with a full-time practice, hospital rounds, on-call duties every other night and every other weekend, community service lectures, and teaching lectures still needs to find four to five spare hours a day in order to write a book. This time would never have been available to me without the devotion and coverage given my patients by my associate, Jay Lamstein, M.D.

The science of nutrition is becoming continuously more sophisticated and developing at a rapid rate. I am especially indebted to three nutritionists who have reviewed my manuscript and have made invaluable contributions to the accuracy and benefits of this book: Margaret B. Salmon, N.S., R.D., A.D.A., director and nutritional consultant of Salmon Consultants, 435 Lynn Street, Harrington Park, New Jersey 07640; Dr. Ronald Drucker, D.C., colleague and nutritional consultant in my office; and Linda Georgian, nutritionist, hostess of the Linda Georgian TV Show (of which I have the honor and privilege to be cohost and medical director).

The difficult task of typing the original manuscript and the many subsequent revisions involved conferences and telephone calls, most of which took place during the evening and on weekends. For her patience, understanding, consideration, and exceptionally professional work, I give special thanks to Sandra Morton.

Finally, to my patients, thank you for your trust, devotion, cooperation, and suggestions; they made the Pleasure Principle a reality for all of us.

                                                    R. E. Willner, M.D.

Contents

The
Pleasure Principle Diet

PROLOGUE
HOW TO LOSE WEIGHT
EATING THE FOODS
YOU LOVE

When you face the facts, life begins.

Do you want the best of all possible worlds?
So do I!

Would you like to be slender and happy?
I'm with you!

Do you want to lose weight eating the foods you love and enjoying your life?
Right on!

Do you want to keep the weight off and eat like everybody else the rest of your life?
Fantastic!

Do you think it's impossible?
Dead wrong! It is possible and you can do it!

If you have been successful in losing weight before, you will be again! This time, however, you will keep the weight off *permanently*. If you weren't able to lose weight before, here is your chance to be successful doing what you know how to do better than anything else— eating the foods that made you fat!

Question: What Is the Pleasure Principle?

Simply, the Pleasure Principle states that we have enough problems, tragedies, disappointments and deprivation in life; therefore, we are entitled to find *pleasure* in everything we do, including eating. It demonstrates how to do this without giving up favorite foods. *In fact, you must eat the foods that made you fat, even while you lose weight, and continue eating those foods for the rest of your life!*

Question: You are going to try to get me so sick of eating fattening foods that I will have to give them up. Right?

Wrong! If you try that stunt, you will end up weighing 600 or 700

1

pounds and will die! *All foods can be fattening,* if you eat enough of them. *No food is fattening,* if the amount you eat doesn't exceed the amount you burn up. Only foods that may be detrimental to health should be avoided.

Question: Then what's the gimmick?

The "gimmick" is to train you to be a "Superstar of Pleasure." Your pleasure, your way of eating, *not* mine or anybody else's. Your own diet! Your own way of life! Your own thing! Your own pleasure!

Question: But my thing got me fat; what changes that?

If you become a superstar, an expert in anything, then you do it better than anyone else. You enjoy it more, and most important, you do it safely and with ease.

Question: How fast can I lose weight?

As fast as your body can safely do it. Faster would be dangerous and deceptive.

Question: What do I have to do?

Invest five minutes a day while you are eating. It doesn't take time away from anything else you want to do.

Question: What do I have to do during those five minutes?

I thought you'd never ask!

THE PLEASURE PRINCIPLE

Some of you must be tired of losing weight and gaining it back, over and over again. You must be tired of restrictive diets that become boring and don't keep your weight off. Would you like to lose weight eating the foods that made you fat? Would you like to continue eating these foods the rest of your life and not have to worry about ever becoming fat again? Well, you can, and that's what this book is all about. The Pleasure Principle offers you a way of accomplishing this with an investment of only five minutes a day. That's all it takes. The method that I am going to outline for you has been used successfully on thousands of patients. *It is as much as forty times better than other methods in keeping weight off.* A six-year office study supports that statement.*

The Pleasure Principle is a positive method. By *positive* I mean that you will not be told that you are forbidden to eat particular foods. In

---

*Government statistics revealed that 98% gained back weight in two years, regardless of the diet used. That is 2% success. My study results showed 80% kept the weight off for six years. Conservatively, that is forty times better.

fact, I insist that you eat the foods that you love. You will be taught a simple system by which you can determine the amount of energy you burn up and the amount of energy you take in; as long as you take in less energy than you burn up, you will lose weight. I have devised a unit of energy that I call the Pleasure Unit. You will be able to look at a plate and, without weighing or measuring the food, quickly estimate the number of Pleasure Units that you will be eating. You can make this estimate right at the table, using any writing implement and any handy piece of paper. This is one of the three rules you *must* follow in the Pleasure Principle. It is the *most important* and it will work for you. Can you honestly say that you can't be bothered? Is five minutes a day too much to ask for the benefits I've promised? If your answer is yes, then you don't want to lose weight; you want somebody else to lose it for you.

Another rule is that you must eat the foods that made you fat. Now that certainly isn't too much to ask. You have been doing it already! This rule will help you lose weight at a reasonable rate, one that is safe and comfortable for you. Start learning to live with pleasure each day, free from guilt and free from irritating restrictions. You must only avoid consuming those foods that are harmful to you, and if you want to lose weight, you must eat less than you burn up. Therefore, *you* regulate the rate at which you lose weight, but it will be easy because of the very simple method I have created. I will recommend to you an intake of between 1000 and 1500 Pleasure Units a day. However, you can increase the amount above 1500 units by earning Pleasure Credits.

Pleasure Credits are the Pleasure Units that you can earn each day in a pleasurable way so that you can spend them on food, or choose not to spend them and lose weight faster. Either way, they will bring you more pleasure. This is an added bonus. If you don't like to do exercise, the Pleasure Principle shows you how enjoying your life can take the place of exercise. It shows you how by increasing the amount of pleasure you get out of life, you can lose weight faster and stay healthier. What could be better than that? You eat what you want to eat! You really know what you're doing, and as you're losing weight you become an expert in recognizing the value of food so well that you can't go off the deep end ever again.

It is not difficult to learn Pleasure Units and Pleasure Credits. You eat between fifty and seventy-five different foods, ninety-nine percent of the time. It won't take you long to learn the Pleasure Units as well as you know your own name and telephone number. At most, there will be only a dozen Pleasure Credits that you will learn, and they, too, will become an automatic part of your thinking.

I've written this book in such a way that you can become an expert in enjoying life, in your knowledge of obesity, in your ability to be a gourmet eater, to lose weight, and to stay thin. If I were to present nothing but a new, exciting method of losing weight, I would be giving you only half of what you should have to ensure success. Your self-understanding will extend the effects of the Pleasure Principle into every part of your life. The first part of the book deals with foods, how the body works, and why fad diets are a waste of time. Virtually every book that has been written about so-called revolutionary diets has included information of this sort. I think I have presented it in a way that is clear, fascinating, and educational. Don't study it, just read it through, but read it! It will make you a better, brighter human being. There are several chapters that deal with the most important person in the world—you! These chapters will help you understand and cope with your feelings. They will assist you in changing your life. I know you want to start losing weight immediately, but do it right! A few hours spent reading the book in sequence will prove to be a valuable and enjoyable investment. When you get to the *"Pleasure Principle,"* I will thoroughly explain this easy, enjoyable way of being a pleasure person. Are you ready for an exciting adventure? Are you ready to give up on the miracle diets that promise, but fail to deliver? Are you ready for a method that stands a forty-times better chance of succeeding where all other methods have failed? If so, become a pleasure person.

I have often thought of the many medical meetings taking place throughout the world each year in which thousands of doctors gather to listen to well-educated, well-motivated, honest, sincere clinicians who praise the basic health principles of a low calorie, well-balanced diet, an exercise program, and emotional support for patients. After all of those hours of repetitious presentations of the same material, which the doctors and the patients already know, the results have not changed: *two percent success.* You would think that somewhere along the line one of my learned colleagues would get up before a thousand or more doctors and say, "Gentlemen, it's all been said before, so I've had it typed up and distributed to you. I would like to spend the next hour asking you if *you* have some *better* suggestions for achieving *results* with our patients!"

Where, then, is the answer? There is a clue in the age-old proverb, "If you can't beat 'em, join 'em." This doesn't mean that every doctor in the country should start joining patients by overeating. It does mean that we should accept reality and work the solution around fact, not wishful thinking.

Some doctors have given up treating patients for obesity because so many of their patients do not succeed in losing weight. I, too, have had patients swear on a stack of bibles that they stuck to their diets and didn't lose an ounce. There is no question that there may be some disturbances in the biochemistry and physiology of the body that make it more difficult for one individual to lose weight than another. All doctors who have dealt with the problem of obesity have observed this unequal, unfair state of events. Sometimes we get the feeling that certain patients are creating carbohydrates from just breathing the carbon, hydrogen, and oxygen out of the air.

Many theories have been proposed to explain why some hungry individuals are quickly satiated after a few bites of food while others are still hungry after finishing a whole plate. The theorists talk about the centers of the brain and the levels of glucose, amino acids, and fats in the blood, and the rate at which they are utilized. The specific dynamic action of ingested food and even body temperature have been studied. Certainly minor variations in each of these influencing factors will cause one individual to respond differently than another. Someone once calculated that a person who eats one doughnut a day in excess of the daily caloric burn would gain 400 pounds of fat over a period of thirty years.

The final answers will be complicated, but we cannot afford to wait for those final answers, because they may not be discovered in our lifetime. The important question is, How do we lose weight *now* in a way in which the benefits far outweigh the disadvantages? More important than that, how can we increase the chances of maintaining that weight loss permanently? No diet program offered up until this very moment has been successful to any reasonable degree. This unfortunately, includes legitimate, well-structured, well-advised, healthy diets. Regretfully, I say to these dedicated, decent professionals, "Your cause is just, your methods are right, but your followers drop by the wayside in such large numbers that you walk alone. Your theory is correct, but no one wants to practice it."

Most of the diet clubs teach sound basic principles of dieting, but their long-term success rate has been only slightly better than that of the individual practitioner. In fact, one of the largest groups won't even make their statistics public. I think that if they did, nobody would attend their meetings. Let's face it, almost any method is going to work for someone. One group has some of its members referring to Chinese beansprouts and diet tomato sauce as "spaghetti"! They even refer to well-done, dried mushrooms as nuts. Can you imagine sitting in front of someone who has a plate of real spaghetti and telling him that your beansprouts and diet tomato sauce are just as good?

One of the most difficult things about dieting is that it tends to isolate the dieter from many other activities. Unless your friends are also on a diet, it is almost impossible to go out with them for dinner. The tendency is to avoid dinner appointments and socialization. It's bad enough when you feel like a food freak, but it is even worse when you have to feel like a social outcast. Very often loneliness itself is the major cause of overeating.

Too many diets stress the negative aspects of living, the concept of denial. Look at some of our severe diabetic patients. For years we have instructed them to maintain a very specific, proportional intake. Their lives are at stake! They face impotence, the loss of their eyesight, gangrene, or premature death, and yet they rarely, if ever, will follow the diet prescribed.

What about starvation or protein diets? Well, losing weight rapidly by starvation or extreme diet plans can have devastating effects. Sexual drive, overall activity, the heart beat, and the level of body metabolism all decrease. Complaints of dizziness or loss of balance and an inability to tolerate heat and cold are very common. These changes reflect the body's attempt to counteract the stress on and deterioration and destruction of the body and its functions caused by such harsh approaches to losing weight. Weight may be lost, but the act of living, the enjoyment of life, and the physiology of the body are all seriously disturbed. In addition to these effects, psychological symptoms also appear. Behavioral changes, depression, irritability, anxiety, hostility, and distortions in perception and feeling usually occur. The importance of food becomes exaggerated, and a sense of being socially isolated as well as deprived is a common experience.

How do I motivate my patients? I first ask them if they really believe in magic, if they are looking for another fad or magical solution. I then ask them if they want to remain children in an adult world, or if they would rather gain a sense of positiveness, of responsibility, of acting and accomplishing. I ask them if they want to live in a real world in a pleasurable way. It is their choice. I try to get my patients to find something good in every moment of each day, to enjoy food more than ever before, run their own lives, and protect, heal, and improve the most important thing in the world—themselves . . . and usually, it works.

THE PLAYBILL
(of Pleasure)

All the world's a stage, and all the men and women merely players. (Shakespeare)

Let me set the stage for you. The single most common, difficult, and destructive problem in medicine is obesity. It is a condition that is incurable, but it can be controlled. During the past twenty years that I have practiced medicine, hundreds of diet programs have been presented as the panacea for this problem. I know them well, because I think I have tried all of them, either on myself or on my patients. Every method that I tried achieved success on a reasonable number of patients. Some methods proved to be relatively safe and others relatively dangerous, but *only two percent of those who lost weight were able to keep it off for more than two years.* This statistic applies to all methods of dieting. My present approach evolved from years of frustration, experimentation, and contact with this wide variety of diets. Is the title for real? You bet your double chin it is!

I have set the stage for this book as one would a play, with a Prologue, Acts, Scenes, and an Epilogue. The reason I chose this format is to stress the importance of your reading it in sequence as you would any play or novel. It follows a logical flow of ideas and concepts that lead to a logical conclusion, starting with what I believe to be a logical premise. If only two percent of all dieters keep their weight off for more than two years, then all the methods that have been used are failures. If all methods have failed, then why do we persist in pursuing the paths that lead to such dismal destinations?

The title of this book was designed to catch your attention, but it is not misleading, *it is not a pitch.* It is, in fact, the method that I advocate and use, and I am sure you will agree it is a method that makes sense. It is safe and provides a most reasonable answer to your problem. I believe that the Pleasure Principle will work for you better than anything else you have tried. Nobody likes to be restricted or deprived. I have excluded the word *calories* from the vocabulary of the Pleasure Principle. Calories are cumbersome, difficult to remember, and almost impossible

7

to use correctly unless you walk around with a scale or a ruler. I do not use the word *exercise* because that word, too, indicates work and an unpleasant activity for most people. The exclusion of words does not mean that I intend to deceive you with semantics. Instead, the words and the concepts associated with them have been excluded from the book because they are negative, negative in concept, or in practice, or through use.

The Pleasure Principle is a positive plan with positive ideas, positive methods, and positive long-term results. By using the Pleasure Principle, you can actually lose weight eating the foods that made you fat, and in fact, *you must eat the foods that made you fat* while you are losing weight in order for it to be effective.

You may be obese, but do you really know what that means? You may feel it, you may live with it each day and be miserable because of it, but do you understand it? It is your enemy and you want to destroy it. You must know your enemy, you must understand it, know where it comes from, what it looks like, and where it is going.

In Scene 1, "Obesity and Overweight," our villian, Obesity, is introduced to you from all perspectives. His weapon is food, particularly the food that you eat, the food that you love, as described carefully in Scene 2, "Food—More Than Just a Mouthful!" This is so important because if we can take these weapons from the villian and use them to our own advantage, then our tale is more likely to end on a note of happiness. Food is also a part of the love interest in the story. The success of the "love affair" depends upon how good a lover our hero (heroine) is, and you will see as the plot develops and thickens that our main character, you—our hero, our heroine—become an expert in love. Everyone knows that love conquers all.

In Scene 3, "Metabolism—the Magnificent Mystifying Machine," the intricacies of the love affair are explored. We will find out what happens to those foods that are taken into your body and how they can help or hurt you. Once you are aware of how the body works, you will feel more secure knowing that the process is going on as it should, and will notice immediately if some kind of a breakdown occurs. The breakdowns and pitfalls are explored in Scene 4, when "Obesity—the 'Mother' of Many Diseases" demonstrates the diabolical tortures awaiting those who fall prey to the enemy's devious ways.

Act I of this play of life covers all of these subjects in a clear and understandable way. It establishes the relationship between you, obesity, and disease, so that being forewarned is being forearmed and, therefore, helps establish the motivation for losing weight.

Without pause, we enter Act II. In Scene 1 we witness the valiant and not so valiant acts of your allies as they endeavor to assist you in defeating your disguised enemies. "In Search of the Truth" (Act II) delves into the promised "Magic, Myths, and Miracles" (Scene 1) that never materialize, or if they do, turn out to be fleeting mirages, temporary crutches, or transient tantalizers. The popular diets of the past few decades are examined for their facts and fallacies, for as you prepare to go into battle, only the most trusted must be at your side. Then, by discarding all other doubtful plans, you embark on a true course.

During the last hours before the battle, we must search for truth in ourselves. "Fuel for Thought" (Scene 2) probes the more common reasons, hidden and obvious, that we overeat and points the way to understanding, controlling, and changing the destructive drives which compel us to destroy ourselves. The last scene of the second act, "The Only Way to Go—Down!," points clearly down the road to success, making the battle imminent and inevitable.

At this moment, at the edge of the climax of the play, the "Intermission" allows us a TIME FOR DECISION, a moment of quiet, a moment for prayer, a moment for contemplation, a moment for meditation. Will you—armed with all of the facts, with the plot tastefully developed, the moment of battle at hand—leave the theater, turn your back on the play, and abandon your quest? Or will you stay. Will you see your way through the entire third act until the conclusion?

The Pleasure Principle unfolds for you in Act III. Armed with understanding, knowledge, and truth we can now actively achieve our goals. In Scene 1, "Pleasure—Real and Deceptive," the plan unfolds, the enemy puts up deceptive targets. The main target is real pleasure; therefore, we must learn to separate it from deceptive pleasure. Deceptive pleasure is not pleasure; it is pain and misery. As in any battle, goals fall into several categories, "Limited, Unlimited, Self-Limited" (Scene 2). When we recognize these categories of pleasure, they never fall short of our expectation; they fill our lives in appropriate ways, making them most fulfilling.

Suddenly, we discover a marvelous revelation. The battle is not arduous, it is not painful, and there are no casualties, except on the opposing side. Our forces are divided into units. The reaching of goals earns more units of pleasure, and it is exciting to discover "Pleasure Begets Pleasure," (Scene 3). The investment in pleasure yields dividends of more pleasure, and those dividends, in turn, propagate further. As the glorious battle develops, we refine the technique of achieving pleasure and enjoy it more.

As victories are won and the successful conclusion draws near, reinforcements are brought up to the edge of the stage, there to be called upon, if needed. Scene 5, "Pleasure Aids—A Helping Hand," offers extra support, something for everyone, to help ensure success. Then, in the end, a total awakening, a firm grip on the future, as you start on your new adventure of life . . . a new hero (heroine), a new being.

THE CURTAIN RISES!

ACT I
UNDERSTANDING OBESITY

A little knowledge is a wondrous thing.

Scene 1
Obesity and Overweight

If we have too much energy stored in our bodies (obesity), it is like a house that is filled up with coal, not just in the basement but in the kitchen, the living room, the bedrooms, in fact, in every room. This leaves no place to live or to enjoy oneself. Isn't this true about obese people? Do they really live and enjoy themselves?

It is estimated that one out of every three Americans is obese. That means that over seventy million Americans weigh more than they should.

WHAT IS OVERWEIGHT? WHAT IS OBESITY?

I recently read an article in one of the medical journals in which over 600 doctors replied to a questionnaire on weight reduction. In response to a question which asked, "When do you consider a patient to be slightly overweight?", answers ranged from five to thirty pounds over the ideal weight. The range for being "seriously overweight" was from ten to one hundred pounds.

Unfortunately, there is no one definition of obesity. The definition of obesity differs from one authority to another. The percentage that you weigh more than your ideal weight will vary from ten to thirty percent depending upon the authority. Patients' perceptions or ideas of what obesity is varies with their ethnic background, social status, educational status, aesthetic values, and personal preference.

Obesity means you're overweight—plain and simple!

In a nutshell, the term *overweight* is a statement of statistical fact. Individuals may be overweight if they compare their frames and weights to those given on the standard charts. They may be overweight because of increased muscle mass, as in the case of athletes, or they may have greater bone size and density, or their bodies may even retain extra fluid.

11

Obesity, however, is more selective in its connotation. It refers to an excessive amount of fat or adipose tissue.

You may have heard the term *morbid obesity*. It is applied to individuals who are at least one hundred pounds overweight or are more than twice the weight indicated on the standard charts.

ARE YOU OBESE?

The following conversation, with many minor variations, has occurred in my office almost daily in the years I have been in practice:

Patient: Doctor, what should I weigh?

Doctor: Well, as a general rule of thumb, a woman who is five feet tall should weigh approximately one hundred pounds. For every inch above five feet, add five pounds

Patient: I am five feet, two inches, Doctor.

Doctor: That means you should weigh approximately 110 pounds.

Patient: But Doctor, I haven't weighed that little since high school.

Doctor: Well, you have been overweight since high school.

In some instances, the condition of overweight is a state of mind rather than a state of being. I have had patients walk into the office with splendid figures (mostly women) and want to be ten, twenty, or even twenty-five pounds below their ideal weight. When they state that they've come into the office to lose weight, I ask, "In which earlobe?" For a very few, the request is a legitimate one and is usually because they do photographic modeling or modeling of some sort. Others request it for emotional reasons.

It is truly amazing how differently individuals see themselves. There are probably many overweight people who should be reading this book, but they don't see themselves that way. Experience has taught me that most individuals do not recognize how fat they really are; there is always a tendency to underestimate the degree of obesity. Even when we judge others, we have a tendency to do the same. Our judgment is often affected by our feelings toward them. If we like someone, we often excuse his state of corpulence by saying that he is pleasingly plump. If, however, we dislike him, we exclaim, "Wow! Is he fat!"

The most difficult people to convince are first-generation Americans because many of them come from cultures where obesity was considered attractive and often reflected wealth.

In past centuries, obesity was a sign of wealth because only the wealthy could afford to eat enough to become obese. Today, the poor also have a tendency to be obese and one wonders whether, in some instances, this is an overcompensation for the fear of doing without. Nevertheless, our society has developed other identifications and other methods of encouraging obesity. Did you ever try to watch television for one hour without seeing advertisements about food? How about magazines? Very often, on the page opposite an article about dieting there will be an ad about some delicious food, complete with mouth-watering pictures.

People and scales are wonderful things. When you put them together, the strangest things happen. When you keep them apart, even stranger things happen. Let's play candid camera for a minute. Have any of these things ever happened to you?

Take Joe the Glut. Now Joe the Glut didn't look at a scale for months or even years on end. Then one day one of his friends said, "Hey Joe, you're getting fat."

A wedding came up and he couldn't get into his old tuxedo. Later, Uncle Charlie died (Charlie weighed 300 pounds) and Aunt Sofie (Charlie's wife) was overheard telling the family that the doctor said that Charlie's weight would be the death of him.

Our friend Joe pulled his car out of the funeral procession on the way to the cemetery to stop off at a drug store and weigh himself. He made it to the cemetery just in time to hear that line about "ashes to ashes, dust to dust."

Joe checked out the bathroom scale when he got home and then the scale down at the men's room in the pool parlor that night. He compared that one with the big scale on the train station the next morning, ran over to the doctor's office at noon time and asked the nurse if he could weigh himself on their scale. Joe weighed himself thirty times that day, and the candid camera caught glimpses of him at each stop. You wouldn't believe the changes in Joe's expression as one scale showed him two pounds more, and another, three pounds less. One scale made him change his expression twenty times because the needle on the dial labored back and forth with each breath and with each movement of the big toe on his left foot. Our friend Joe got tired of looking for coins every time he wanted to weigh himself and finally bought a portable scale which he carried in his attaché case. When last heard from, Joe had set a new world's record for the "Greatest Number of Times Weighed in Twenty-Four Hours." While Joe was a guest at the state mental institution in Room 244-B, the walls were covered with the strangest numbers: $262\frac{1}{2}$, $262\frac{3}{8}$, $264\frac{1}{4}$, $265\frac{1}{6}$ . . .

Of course, you bear no resemblance to Joe the Glut. However, to prevent any misunderstanding, let me give you some good ideas that will help you lose weight and not your sanity.

WEIGHING YOURSELF DAILY

Zeal without knowledge,
is a fire without a light.

The importance of weighing yourself daily is in learning how the body functions and verifies the metabolic process described in this book. You will note that the weight loss is rarely steady. In fact, it may even go up a pound when you have expected it to go down. When you have followed the Pleasure Principle, you will know that you *must* be losing fat, even though it doesn't show on the scale. It is best to evaluate the actual weight loss on a weekly basis, but if you get into the habit of weighing yourself daily and do it regularly, just as you brush your teeth every morning, you then are facing reality and not turning your back on your problem. How many times have you said, "I can't bear to look in the mirror," or, "I can't bear to look at the scale," or, "I don't want to look at the scale today because I know I've gained weight."? It would be far healthier, on those troublesome days, to reaffirm your goal or seek help. *The proper way to weigh yourself is in the morning, immediately upon rising and after emptying your bladder.* This gives you a base line each day. Do not weigh yourself again during the day, because even though you're dieting, your weight may go up.

PLATEAUS

Because losing weight is a proportional phenomenon, adjustments of energy intake may have to be made periodically. It has been the experience of most doctors who have treated overweight patients that a patient will periodically hit a plateau, a point at which weight loss seems to stop for a period of several days or even several weeks. The body seems to resist losing weight at these points, and even though the patients religiously stick to the diet, they fail to lose weight. A reduction in energy intake and/or an increase in energy output must be made in order to help some of these patients. The reasons for this occurrence are not well understood. Suffice it to say that you may have to accept the fact that you will reach your ultimate goal a few weeks later.

The concept of homeostasis has long been observed in medicine. It basically refers to the tendency of the body to maintain its current state, to resist change. The process of losing weight is not a smooth one because many things are going on at the same time and at different rates, and there is much evidence to indicate that the body shifts gears in an attempt to fight stress and great changes. This is accomplished through hormone and enzyme systems that will be discussed at length in the chapter on metabolism.

The weight reflected on a scale represents many factors that fall into two categories:

1. Long-term mass and weight. The long-term factors include your bone, muscle, and most of your body tissue.

2. Short-term mass and weight. The short-term factors include the food in your stomach and intestines, the waste material in the intestines, the fluids flowing through the body and present in hollow organs, such as the intestines and the bladder, and even the perspiration on the skin, the air in your lungs, and the temporary water retained in the cells of your body, such as that which causes bellies to bloat, rings to fit tight on fingers, and feet to swell at night.

During weight loss, water may be retained for as long as three weeks. Salt or high carbohydrate meals encourage water retention. Unless you are extremely uncomfortable it is unwise to take a diuretic (water pill) and best to just keep on your program of losing weight. *It may not be showing on the scale, but you must be losing weight if you are burning up more than you are taking in.* The reason it doesn't show up on the scale is that the waste products may be in transit, either in the blood stream, in the tissue spaces, in the bowels, or in the bladder. The rate of weight loss is different for everyone, so never compare yourself to someone else. If you stick to your plan, you must be burning up the fat. In order to push past a plateau you might try a "unifood day." Choose only one of the following foods—apples, cantaloupe, or grapefruit—and eat only that food plus water for one day.

Insurance companies have been of great service to the public in the field of health. They have provided us with information that has allowed us to establish standards for normality and to understand the risk of disease.

An incredible amount of time and effort has gone into the collection of data on millions of individuals in order to come up with the standard weight charts that health professionals use today. Weight tables are averages and serve as guides for determining the ideal weight for most people. They take into consideration your height and your frame. Your frame is determined by body structure. If your body structure has been covered up by fat for a long period of time, it might be rather difficult to determine what classification you fall into. In fact, it has been my experience that most individuals have a tendency to describe their frames as larger than they actually are. Another complication in determining frame size is the variation that occurs in body proportions. Some individuals have broad frames in the area of the shoulders but are very narrow in the area of the hips. Others may be just the opposite. I use the charts to help a patient reach a level of weight close to the middle of the large frame. When they reach that point, I then reevaluate how they look and take measurements which help determine how much more they should lose. In reality, most individuals fall into the small and medium frame categories.

Some men and women, particularly athletes, or those engaged in careers that primarily involve physical activity, may be overweight according to standard tables, but they are not obese. Obese individuals have an abundance of fat tissue. Obviously then, the scale doesn't tell the whole story. Although an overweight person may not be obese, obese people are usually overweight, and some of normal weight may be obese.

One technique the physician will often use to assess the amount of fat present on the body is the caliper test. The caliper is a simple instrument used to measure the thickness of a fold of skin, not muscle, in those areas where fat usually accumulates. A simple "home" method for doing your own caliper test is to pick up a fold of skin on the side of your waist, or near the bottom of your chest (toward one side), on the back of your upper arms, or on your thigh.

Don't pinch hard, just gently pick it up.

If the thickness is approximately an inch or more, you are probably obese. The area most frequently used in medicine to measure the skin fold thickness is the fat tissue overlying the triceps muscle. This is located on the back of your arm halfway between your elbow and your shoulder.

Rather than depend upon your own prejudiced point of view as to what weight is normal for you, I strongly suggest that you use the chart I've included in this chapter to determine what that weight should be. Remember, too, that you have to try to judge your body build honestly. Is your frame small, medium, or large? If you have any doubt, you should consider your frame medium and aim for the lower figure in that range. If you are still not sure about your frame, try this:

Wrap the thumb and middle finger of your left hand around your right wrist. If your fingers do not touch, you have a large frame. If your fingers touch, you have a medium frame. If your fingers overlap, you have a small frame. (If you are left handed, measure your left wrist with your right hand.)

When you have finally reached your listed ideal weight, there is an additional method that you can use to test the accuracy of the chart.

Strip down and stand in front of the mirror.

Don't ask yourself if you are fat, because if you do, you would probably answer, "I'm not so fat."

Better questions would be "Is that the figure I have always wanted?" "Do I like the way I look?" "Would someone of the opposite sex like the way I look?"

The answer has got to be yes or no, not, "Well, it's close" or "it's not so bad." Just answer yes or no!

Now, stop looking just at your face!

Look all the way down, don't be embarrassed! I don't want to know if there are some things that should be smaller and other things that should be bigger.

Now cut it out, stop pulling yourself in!

Just stand relaxed.

You're still having trouble? Let me give you a couple of hints. Look at your cheeks, your chin, your breasts, the area in front of your armpits, your belly, your waist on the sides, your buttocks, your thighs. If your answer is yes, you like what you see, then there are two possibilities: (1) You're obviously not reading this book because you're overweight, but just curious about the Pleasure Principle, and if so, read on, dear friend. (2) You need a consultation from a psychiatrist or an ophthalmologist.

If your answer is no, you don't like what you see, then you are overweight. Join the fellow who is curious about the Pleasure Principle.

For purposes of classification, medicine has categorized human beings into three body types: the ectomorph, who is usually slender; the meso-morph, who is usually more of the muscular type; and the endomorph, who is typically heavyset. These classifications are actually related not only to body structure but to the way that we think and feel. There is a fairly strong correlation between the frame and the individual's person-ality.

While researching this book, I came across a description of the ectomorph as a fragile individual who likes to be by himself, is studious, has trouble sleeping, is sensitive to pain, is embarrassed easily, and does not care for routine. The mesomorph was described as being bold, active, full of energy, youthful, and fond of physical competition. The endo-morph was listed as a talkative, foodloving, sentimental, self-satisfied individual who sleeps quite well. There is probably some truth to all this, but one must wonder which came first, the chicken or the egg? Did these behavioral and emotional characteristics lead people to develop distinctive physical statures? Did the genetic body type cause society to react to each growing child in such a manner that the emotional characteristics developed as they did? Or was everything genetically determined? We all can think of a few jovial fat people who have been the life of the party. I can also remember some of them coming into my office desperately seeking help to escape from the prison of fat in which they were enclosed. The jolly personality was only a cover up, a means of attracting the attention and friendship of others in what was otherwise a very lonely, uncomfortable, unhappy existence. I have never met a truly happy fat person, and I have met very few *old* ones.

Obviously, genetics does play a role in limiting our objectives. In terms of the real world that we live in, genetics simply means that your idealized goal of how you would like to look may not be totally achieved because of inherited characteristics. In obesity, the ratio of fat tissue to all the other tissues of the body is increased. The skin folds of the body and the total body mass are oversized. The distribution of fat cells follows a genetic or family pattern, and if there is a particular fat deposit area on your body that continues to have a larger mass or size than you would like after you have brought your weight down into normal range, then the only suitable solution may be plastic surgery or aspiration of fat.

If your frame is not to your liking, you face a more difficult problem. For example, if you would like to have slender hips, the size to which you can reduce them may be limited by the bony structure underneath, and there is no way that you can reduce bone, except by surgery. I strongly advise against such surgery except under the most unusual circumstances (a common exception, however, would be a rhinoplasty, or plastic surgery of the nose, where bone is often partially removed). You would be far better off to aim for a proportional body that is pleasing to the eye rather than thinking in terms of a perfect figure, whatever that is. Accept what nature has given you, but make the very best of it.

I'M FAT—NOW WHAT?

If you are obese, the decision to lose weight is a good one. The way in which you lose it, however, may be bad. I would like you to consider yourself in the same way in which I consider you. You are the most important person in the world. Unless you are well trained in auto mechanics, I wouldn't suggest that you tamper with your car; similarly, unless you are a physician, I don't recommend that you tamper with your body without expert advice. Although you will gain a good basic knowledge of obesity and body metabolism and learn a sound approach to losing weight by reading this book, I strongly advise that you get a

DESIRABLE WEIGHTS

(Based on Height and Body Frame)*

Height		Small	Medium	Large
Feet	Inches	Frame	Frame	Frame
4	10	92–98	96–107	104–119
4	11	94–101	98–110	106–122
5	0	96–104	101–113	109–125
5	1	99–107	104–116	112–128
5	2	102–110	107–119	115–131
5	3	105–113	110–122	118–134
5	4	108–116	113–126	121–138
5	5	111–119	116–130	125–142
5	6	114–123	120–135	129–146
5	7	118–127	124–139	133–150
5	8	122–131	128–143	137–154
5	9	126–135	132–147	141–158
5	10	130–140	136–151	145–163
5	11	133–144	140–155	149–168
6	0	138–148	144–159	153–173

Women

*Based on Metropolitan Life Insurance Company, Tables of Desirable Weight.

good general checkup from your doctor and enlist his or her supervision during the time that you are losing weight, especially if you intend to lose more than 10% of your body weight. There are many conditions which may need monitoring in order for you to accomplish your goal. Even though you are sure you are healthy, you will feel a lot better if an expert confirms it. You may have an early reversible stage of one of the diseases often associated with obesity. Even if the condition is not reversible it is most likely controllable, and in that case the physician's assistance is doubly imperative.

As you learn more about food and body metabolism you will understand why a physical checkup and a periodic follow-up by a physician is necessary. If your physician does not choose to handle the problem, ask him to recommend a bariatrician, a specialist in obesity problems. Beware of the bariatrician who insists on your going through a whole new battery of blood tests, EKGs, and chest X-rays when you have had

DESIRABLE WEIGHTS

(Based on Height and Body Frame)*

Men

Height Feet	Inches	Small Frame	Medium Frame	Large Frame
5	2	112–120	118–129	126–141
5	3	115–123	121–133	129–144
5	4	118–126	124–136	132–148
5	5	121–129	127–139	135–152
5	6	124–133	130–143	138–156
5	7	128–137	134–147	142–161
5	8	132–141	138–152	147–166
5	9	136–145	142–156	151–170
5	10	140–150	146–160	155–174
5	11	144–154	150–165	159–179
6	0	148–158	154–170	164–184
6	1	152–162	158–175	168–189
6	2	156–167	162–180	173–194
6	3	160–171	167–185	178–199
6	4	164–175	172–190	182–204

*Based on Metropolitan Life Insurance Company, Tables of Desirable Weights.

them done within the last six months by your own doctor. Instead, he should ask to review the tests you have already had done and, of course, do his own physical examination. Most important, he should ask for a complete medical history, including a detailed emotional history, and thoroughly investigate your eating habits. I have provided a sample history form for your reference. (page 21).

Unexplained weight gain or weight loss, particularly if unexpected, can be significant. You would probably be overjoyed to get on the scale and find that you have lost weight, especially if you are fat. However, if this weight loss cannot be explained by the fact that you have eaten less or have been far more active than usual, then it could be a symptom of a hidden disease. Loss of appetite or change in bowel habits should always be looked upon with suspicion. The medical definition of diarrhea is a softening of the consistency and/or an increase in the number of bowel

OBESITY HISTORY

Name_____Age_____Height_____Weight_____
Occupation_____Religion_____
Nationality_____Last grade attended in school_____
Weight you would like to be_____
How much weight would you like to lose?_____
What's the highest weight you have ever weighed?_____
   How old were you?_____
What members of your family have been obese?_____
Approx. how many times have you been on a diet in your life?_____
List the diets_____
_____

How long have you been overweight?_____
What is the least you have weighed and when?_____
What is the most you have lost in the shortest period of time?:
   Pounds_____Inches_____Weeks_____Months_____Years_____
After the last time you dieted, what was the least you weighed?_____
How much did you lose while on your last diet?_____
Why do you think you are overweight?_____

How many times a day do you eat?_____
Number of meals?_____Number of snacks?_____
What percentage of the time do you usually eat at:
   Home_____Restaurants_____Social occasions_____
At what time do you start work?_____How many hours do you work?___
What exercise do you do?_____

What activities do you *like* to do?_____
Do you eat when you are depressed or anxious?_____
Do you eat in response to any other emotional feelings?_____
   If yes, describe_____

Describe the meals and snacks that you eat on a typical day_____
_____
_____

Do you feel this is a balanced diet?_____
What do you think a balanced diet means?_____

Do you eat more on weekends and holidays?_____
Do you usually finish all the food on your plate?_____
Do you take extra helpings?_____How much?_____
Do you eat bread or rolls?_____How much?_____
What liquids do you usually drink?_____

What foods do you *like* to eat (List all dishes, sandwiches, desserts and candy)

_____

_____

_____

(The above form asks additional questions of the would-be dieter beyond those found in the standard history and physical forms that most doctors use.)

movements. For example, if you ordinarily have a bowel movement every other day and you suddenly have two movements every day, even though they are of normal consistency, this could be a sign that something has gone wrong. On the other hand, if you improve your diet you'll most likely begin to have normal bowel movements. Seek your doctor's help, however, rather than passing it off as a mysterious blessing that is causing you to lose weight.

All of us have had the experience of wanting to "murder" some individuals who seem to be able to eat anything, and as much of it as they like, while staying thin. The answer to this mystery must be one of the following:

1. They don't eat as much as you think, as often as you think.
2. They must be burning up more energy than they are taking in.
3. Their thinness may be a disease state, and although you might not agree, I would rather need to watch my weight than have any of the diseases that could cause that phenomenon.
4. They may be eating a more nutritious diet.

O.K., then tell me, doctor . . .

WHAT CAUSES OBESITY?

The great debate continues, and it has gone on for a long time. What causes obesity? (Choose the appropriate answers.)
Obesity is caused by

( ) Genetics   ( ) The Wrong Food
( ) Habit   ( ) Too Little Exercise
( ) Glandular Disorders   ( ) Economics
( ) Too Much Food   ( ) Social Status
( ) Emotions   ( ) Cultural Background
                    ( ) All of the Above

The answer is that any one, a combination of some, or all of these factors can cause obesity. To the researcher, the physician, and you, it is important to know which factors are responsible in each case—especially in yours! For, if any of these factors are ignored, losing weight can be as difficult as swimming up a waterfall.

In my opinion, the three most common causes of obesity are overeating, inactivity, and eating the wrong foods. Genetic factors and impairment of body functions are far less important. The most common reasons for overeating and physical inactivity are emotional and social factors. These will be discussed at length, later on.

Some of the ominous omens of obesity are:

1. A birth weight greater than nine pounds (this may also be an indication of familial diabetic tendencies)
2. A family history of obesity
3. Being fat in the first ten years of life
4. Growing up in a lower socioeconomic class
5. A history of substantial fluctuations in weight

Recent studies have indicated that childhood obesity is associated with an increased number of fat cells. Related research seems to indicate that if people would restrict calorie intake early in life, they may be able to decrease the number of these fat cells, and the chance of children becoming obese as they grow older may be less. Another interesting observation is that obese children usually become obese adults and obese parents usually have obese children. This seems to indicate that children follow the patterns of their parents. The *distribution* of fat, as well as the *tendency* to become fat, appears to be inherited. Whether or not your state of obesity is due to environment, heredity, or both really makes no difference to your goal of becoming slender, however. People can't change their past, much less their genetic makeup. The job is simply one that has to be done regardless of the relative difficulties it may present.

Physical activity can actually reduce the number of fat cells in fatty tissue. This, unfortunately, appears to be more applicable in early life than in later life. So, even though this fact may have greater bearing on the adolescent than the adult, the activity itself will help burn up calories and reduce the bulk of the fatty tissue. The fat cells in the obese individual are enlarged and, therefore, hold more fat. Obesity, therefore, depends on two factors with regard to the fatty tissue. The number of fat cells and the size or bulk of each fat cell. This does not mean that these factors are the cause of obesity. They may actually be the result of obesity.

Age, is of course, a factor in being overweight, but be careful not to interpret this incorrectly. It does not mean, as so many people think, that as you get older, you should naturally weigh more. On the contrary, if anything, you should weigh less. It does mean, however, that as you get older you will probably be less active and burn up less energy. Consequently, in order to keep your weight where it is, you would have to take in less energy (food) to avoid gaining weight. It is undesirable to be overweight at any age, but more dangerous as you get older, a fact we will explore in the chapter on Obesity and Disease.

Contrary to what you may have heard, activity plays a very significant role in the problem of weight. Walking up a flight of stairs, for instance, consumes twenty times as much energy as resting in bed. It is true that the desire for food increases as the level of physical activity increases, but as the activity level decreases, hunger may not decrease proportionately. Consequently, inactive persons usually take in more energy than they burn up.

Your daily routine plays an important role in determining the amount of energy you can take in, in order to maintain your weight or in order to lose weight, if that be your object. The number of children you have to take care of, the size of the house you have to clean, the kind of a job you have, and the type of recreation you prefer are all significant. The patterns of our lives change too. In the first twenty years of life we use up a lot more energy in our daily physical activity than we do as we get older. Our jobs may involve sitting behind a desk or they may involve doing heavy construction work. All of these factors will have a profound influence on our weight. Naturally, activity and age are interrelated. So even if you kept the same daily routine for forty years, the energy that you burned up on a daily basis would gradually diminish over the years.

Another factor that determines your ideal weight is your socioeconomic position in life. Actors, models, basketball players, football players, wrestlers, and even doctors have to live up to a certain image determined by the requirements of their job. Regardless of the appeal of the method that I present to my patients, I would hardly be convincing if I myself were overweight. Sexual attractiveness is important to most people, but there are two sides to the issue. Your weight may either increase or decrease your sex life. The rabbit has justly earned his reputation by virtue of his ability to make quick moves, but does anyone praise the hippopotamus for his sexual prowess? By utilizing all of the factors presented, the weight charts, the mirror, the scale, your body type, your socioeconomic needs, you will be able to adequately determine what your ideal weight should be—and who is going to argue over a few pounds, more or less?

Women fall victim to obesity in their adult years more than any other group. During this time the tendency to gain weight is greater than at any other in their lives. Women should be alerted to manage their eating habits carefully and promote healthy energy output during adolescence, pregnancy, and menopause.

The pattern of eating—that is, the number of meals a day and the times at which they are eaten—appears to play a role in weight gain and loss. The process of eating itself expends energy, and the tendency to store food is stimulated after long fasts. The evidence is not clear, but for some people, eating smaller meals several times a day reduces the tendency to overeat, as does eating earlier in the day and avoiding late suppers.

Medication can unquestionably play a role in causing obesity. The drugs used today that are most commonly implicated in cases of overweight are the estrogen products, particularly birth control pills. This is the reason so many women have chosen to discontinue the pills and find other means of contraception. If you are taking medication and notice that you are putting on weight, bring up the question with your doctor.

In a discussion of the causes of obesity, endocrine or glandular causes, although very rare, cannot be left out. Physicians know that the glandular causes are rare, but if you listened to the obese patients you would be inclined to believe that glandular problems are the only cause. In our society we are oriented to the idea that a pill will take care of everything. It would be far more consoling to know that you have a disease or condition that could be easily cured, that you can take a small pill and your troubles will be over. At the present time, however, there is no known glandular disease responsible for 99% of the overweight population. You might also consider that when the only symptom that a patient has is obesity, it is extremely unlikely that the patient has a glandular problem. I would like to list the glandular diseases and their common symptoms so you can be reassured that you probably don't have any of them.

DISEASES CAUSING OBESITY

Cushing Syndrome

This disease is often caused by the prolonged use of cortisone and its derivatives and is characterized by obesity, high blood pressure, excess hairiness, purplish stripes on the abdomen, a face that looks like a moon, and a large pad of fat above the collar bones and on the back of the neck, in addition to a tendency to impairment of glucose tolerance (both low and high blood sugars).

Laurence-Moon-Biedl Syndrome

Characterized by obesity, retinitis pigmentosa with visual disturbances, mental retardation with microcephaly (small head), polydactyly (extra fingers or toes), and hypogenitalism (small gonads [testis or ovaries]).

Alstrom Syndrome

Same as above, but no mental retardation or polydactyly. Also present: deafness, kidney disease with diabetes insipidus (frequent urination, production of huge amounts of urine), baldness.

Prader-Labhart-Willi Syndrome

Characterized by obesity, almond-shaped eyes, low-set ears, mental retardation, loss of muscle tone; patient is usually short in stature.

Fröhlich Syndrome

Usually brought about by damage or tumor in the hypothalamus; characterized by obesity, sexual organ dysfunction, diabetes insipidus, uncontrollable appetite.

Hypothyroidism

Among children, a severe case would exhibit mental retardation. The tongue would be large and protruding, the skin and hair coarse, and the voice harsh and low. Bone growth is retarded as is the appearance of teeth. In the adult, fatigue, drowsiness, weakness, hoarseness, intolerance to cold, constipation, dry skin, edema (puffiness of hands and feet extending to the arms and legs), vague aches and pains, unusual sensations in the skin (in medicine called paresthesias), excessive vaginal bleeding, spontaneous habitual abortion, loss of sexual drive, loss of muscle tone, indigestion, belching or passing gas rectally, irritability, and, of course, obesity.

The last disease, hypothyroidism, is the catchall because most of us at one time or another have suffered from some of the symptoms listed. Today, the overwheming majority of cases of hypothyroidism can be diagnosed by means of blood samples and, if necessary, the nuclear techniques of radioactive assays and thyroid scans.

A physician once quipped, "The only gland that is consistently involved in obesity is in the salivary gland, the gland that makes your mouth water."

Now that you know you are *just obese,* let's proceed!

Scene 2
Food—More Than Just a Mouthful

I wish I could figure out Joe the Glut. He got his new car the other day, and after driving it out of the showroom he stopped at a local news stand and bought thirteen magazines about cars. He then drove into a parking lot, parked his car, and started thumbing through all of the advertisements. Pen in hand, he busily checked off ads of all kinds, then quickly ripped them out, put them in a neat pile, and took off again. His next stop was the automobile enthusiast's emporium, where he rolled a shopping cart down fourteen aisles of car accessories. He bought a super gas gismo that sits on the carburetor—guaranteed to save you one tenth of one percent on your gas consumption. He then bought an incredible ignition intensifier, the remarkable emission recycler, the fantastic fuel fabricator, several gadgets that promised to convert water, orange juice, and cod liver oil into gas, and forty assorted cans of gas additives, oil additives, transmission additives, radio additives and additive additives. His bill came to $323.42.

It took Joe seven weekends to put all of these gadgets on his car. The additives were pretty potent; they bubbled up the paint on his fenders and ate deep holes into the asphalt driveway. The outcome of all this was that Joe's super Lincolack got an additional 6.2 mpg of gas over the next year, which amounted to a savings of $26.37 for the year. Joe argued that that sum would amount to considerable savings if he kept his car long enough for it to be an antique. The problem is that Joe trades in his car every year.

You are probably wondering what that story was all about. The point is that Joe was putting all those things in his car without knowing what they were and what they would actually do. Joe reminds me of a lot of people who put various things into their bodies without knowing what will happen either. My object is therefore to make you an expert in your way of life, particularly in regard to your problem of obesity. I'm a great lover of food. If you are like me and you are reading this book, then you must have had some problems with your love affair. A great lover should always try to have a thorough understanding of the object of his love. So, fellow food lovers, how about a little advice for the lovelorn.

In order for your love affair with food to enrich your life rather than destroy it, you have to be an expert. Besides, in order to carry out the Pleasure Principle, you must thoroughly understand and know the foods that you eat. Love usually generates a lot of heat and heat is a form of energy. Similarly, food generates a lot of energy. The unit used to measure the energy value of food is called a *calorie.*

In the Playbill, I told you that we would not use the term *calorie* in the Pleasure Principle, and when you get to the third act it will be abandoned. But first you need to understand what a calorie is and the role it plays in the foods that you eat and in the functioning of your body.

A calorie is defined as the amount of heat required to raise the temperature of one liter of water one degree centigrade. Or, expressed in units that you might be more familiar with, it is the amount of heat needed to raise the temperature of a pint of water four degrees fahrenheit (the temperature measurement used by your thermometer). In terms of food, for example, one level teaspoon of white granulated sugar will yield sixteen calories when burned by your body. All calories are alike regardless of the foods that produce them, but the number of calories generated in the production of energy will vary with the type and amount of food.

The food we eat serves our bodies in two basic ways. First, as a source of energy, food provides the fuel to keep the body going, supporting all of the internal and external functions of the body: the functioning of the brain and of respiratory, intestinal, genito-urinary, and glandular systems as well as the muscular activity that provides us with the ability to move, work, play, and enjoy our lives. Second, it provides the materials necessary to build, repair, maintain, and replace the cells that compose the tissues of all of the different kinds of structures in our bodies.

The human body is composed of four basic substances: water, fat, active cell tissue, and bone. The entire structure is in a constant state of repair and replacement. An estimated five percent of your body weight changes every day. This includes bone, nails, hair, nerves, and all tissues and organs. This process goes on every day of your life. When I hear people say that they are going to go out of this world the same way they came in, I always chuckle.

If someone tells you that you are not the same person today that you were yesterday, you could take that statement literally. So you see, not only does the experience of living change your personality, but your body also changes. The rate of replacement varies for each kind of tissue of the body, and the substances needed to effect this change are of a wide variety. Some of the essential materials are nutrients needed for effecting these changes and can be stored by the body, but others cannot be. Five basic categories of essential nutrients are protein, carbohydrates, fats, vitamins, and minerals. However, food is usually just classified into three basic types: proteins, carbohydrates, and fats. Most foods are made up of combinations of all three of these substances but are categorized according to their main ingredient. For example, beef contains protein and fat, but is called protein. Its composition varies but is in the range of five to one, protein to fat, when lean and of good grade.

Let's take a closer look at these three different types of food.

PROTEIN

Proteins are the basic building blocks of living matter. Protein is, for example, the basic ingredient of muscle. Protein exists in many different forms and differs from one animal species to another, as well as from one plant or vegetable to another. And, here's a surprise for you: bone, the substance which makes up your skeleton, is composed of connective tissue impregnated with calcium and phosphorous compounds. The connective tissue is called collagen, a protein which when boiled down is converted into gelatin.

Protein is the primary substance found in meats, and this variety is referred to as animal protein. Protein is also found in vegetables and fruits, although usually in smaller amounts and referred to as vegetable protein. Proteins are very complex chemical structures composed of separate units called *amino acids*.

Amino acids are made up of carbon, hydrogen, and oxygen, as are carbohydrates, but in addition to these three elements amino acids contain nitrogen. Many proteins also contain phosphorous and sulfur. The number of types of protein that can be made from the twenty-two known amino acids is almost limitless. Each species of animal, each type of tissue, is made up of different proteins.

Proteins may contain all or some of the amino acids in an almost infinite variety of combinations. This, of course, accounts for the incredible varieties of protein found in nature.

Our body is capable of manufacturing twelve out of the twenty-two amino acids. The remaining ten are not manufactured by the body, and it is essential that the body receive these amino acids regularly in the food supply because they are not stored by the body either. These amino acids are therefore referred to as the "essential amino acids." If the body does not obtain any of the essential amino acids, then the protein that depends upon them will not be produced. The constant repair of tissue cannot take place properly and body proteins will be broken down. The protein of the body that cannot have its defective parts replaced can no longer maintain its identity and is destroyed. When this occurs, nitrogen, which is one of the components of amino acid, is released and excreted by the kidney in large amounts, thus creating what is commonly referred to as a negative nitrogen balance and indicating a loss of muscle or protein tissue from the body.

Generally speaking, the diet in the United States contains more than enough protein. Consequently, athletes who take extra protein are merely getting extra energy that could be consumed in any form (fats or carbohydrates) but, unfortunately, creates extra work for the kidneys to do.

Children not fed a sufficient supply of animal protein may become retarded, have growth deficiencies, and develop disease of the blood system and of the liver. The rare protein deficiency diseases are usually found among vegetarians.

There are two types of vegetarians, those that omit and those that include eggs and dairy products. Those that exclude eggs or dairy products should be strongly advised to eat nuts, seeds, and legumes. Aside from being rich in protein, these foods also contain vitamins and minerals. In addition, vegetarians should be encouraged to eat enriched cereals and breads, fruits, and vegetables. Common deficiencies in calcium and vitamin B-12 can be corrected with turnip greens, collard greens, and other dark green vegetables. In order to obtain these vitamins and minerals, as well as vitamin D, vegetarians may require fortified foods or supplements, and by including seaweed or iodized salt in their diet, they will meet their iodine requirements. Vegetables usually do not contain all of the amino acids, and in order to obtain the essential ones, a very wide variety of vegetables must be eaten in sufficient quantities. This is impossible and unhealthy for most persons.

However, in our country it is unusual to see any of the deficiency diseases because the essential amino acids are readily available in foods that are abundant, such as milk, eggs, meat, chicken, and fish.

Protein contains four calories per gram. Translated into a more recognizable entity, a quarter pound hamburger (which also contains fat) would be approximately 225 calories. A strip of bacon, broiled or fried to a crisp so that the fat is rendered out, would be approximately 50 calories. A half-pound sirloin steak has approximately 250 calories.

Don't bother memorizing calories because, as I told you in the Playbill, when you get to "The Pleasure Principle," Act III, we are going to abandon calories and show you an easy way to know what you are doing.

There are only a few common foods that are almost pure protein: scallops, snails, trout, ocean perch, lobster, shrimp, cod, crab, flounder, frogs' legs, haddock, clams, sweetbreads, egg white, and uncreamed cottage cheese (low fat). This is one reason why seafood and eggs are a highly recommended part of your diet.

There are some foods that are ordinarily thought of as being basically protein but have an extremely high content of fat. Cooked hamburger, for example, has almost as much fat as protein, and because *fat has nine calories per gram* as compared to four for protein, most of the calories from the hamburger are coming from the fat. All chicken is not the same, either. For example, when you buy the flesh and skin fryers you're getting protein four to one over fats, but if you purchase a hen the protein and fat are almost equal. Therefore, do not eat the skin. If you eat duck, you're in for a real surprise. The fat is almost twice as much by weight as the protein and, therefore, the caloric value comes from the fat four to one over the protein. Pork chops contain more fat than protein, and when you eat spareribs, it's two to one fat over the proteins. In prepared meats, such as sausages, bologna, and salami, the fat content is even higher; these should not be eaten often or at all.

CARBOHYDRATES

Carbohydrates are made up of carbon, hydrogen, and oxygen (chemical abbreviation C,H, and O). They contain *four calories per gram.* They consist of what are known as simple sugars. Sucrose is the major component of table sugar, fructose is the major component in fruits, and galactose is the sugar found in milk products. In foods, these sugars are not usually found in their simple state; they are usually in combination. For example, table sugar is a chemical combination of glucose and fructose. Milk sugar is a chemical combination of glucose and galactose. Malt sugar is a linking together of two glucose chains.

Starch, of which there are two types, vegetable and animal starch (glycogen), is made up of long chains of glucose molecules. Vegetable starches are found in grains, vegetables, and in fruits. The general misconception is that we can consume starches as sugar, breads, fruit, and cakes, as a substitute for vegetable or animal carbohydrates. They are more likely to affect our weight and health adversely, however, because they are *simple* sugars, and contain few essential nutrients. Animal starch is stored in animal tissue, primarily muscle which we call meat and liver. It is the body's means of storing a quick energy reserve.

Cellulose, which is another carbohydrate, is responsible for the bulk of most fruits and vegetables. It is, in fact, the carbohydrate which is most abundant in fruits and vegetables. It is the substance that forms the food fiber about which we have heard so much in the past few years. It is not digestible by the body because we lack the enzymes that are necessary to break it down into the simpler sugars that can be absorbed. Although cellulose doesn't supply us with energy, it does, however, serve to help us keep our bowels functioning properly by providing the bulk so necessary for regularity. Because it is not absorbed, it does not provide any calories and passes through the body basically untouched. It is one of the reasons that *some* fruits, and especially vegetables can be eaten in large amounts without fear of overdosing yourself with a source of energy.

FATS

Fats are composed of a substance called glycerol, which is linked to three fatty acids. It is for this reason that fats are often referred to as tri-glycerides. Like proteins and carbohydrates, the fatty acids are made up of carbon, hydrogen, and oxygen. The major difference lies in the manner in which these atoms are linked to one another. Characteristically, fatty acids are a chain of carbon atoms to which hydrogen is attached. The shorter the chain of carbon atoms, the more liquid the fat is. The longer the chain, the more solid the fat is. During the past ten years the terms saturated and unsaturated fat have entered the vocabulary of the general public. Many products have been sold through the media as polyunsaturated. What does it all mean? Well, you'll remember that I said that the carbon atoms have hydrogen atoms linked to them. Now, if any of the links to the carbon atom are not taken up by hydrogen, the molecule would be referred to as unsaturated, meaning that it is capable of taking on more hydrogen. If it could take on more than one hydrogen, it would be referred to as poly-unsaturated. Unsaturated fatty acids are more easily burned by the body, but they require additional vitamins A & E in the diet. The polyunsaturated fats are derived from vegetables. The oils that come from safflower, peanut, cotton seed, soy bean, and corn are poly-unsaturated. The fats that are found in poultry, pork, beef, butter, cream, and eggs is saturated fat. The poly-unsaturated fats appear to reduce the amount of cholesterol and fat in the blood stream. The consumption of sugar increases the fat and triglyceride level in the blood stream.

Remember that most foods contain more than one of the three substances I have just described, carbohydrates, proteins, and fats, and that the processing of these foods goes on simultaneously in the body.

VITAMINS

Vitamins are vital and essential in maintaining good health and cannot be synthesized by the body. They are substances present in your food that help your body function normally. Vitamins are involved in the chemical reactions of the body that are responsible for the production of energy, the building of tissue, and the movement and transfer of energy throughout the body. When there is a deficiency or absence of vitamins, these chemical reactions cannot take place properly and the chemicals participating in these reactions would accumulate, causing serious illness which could even lead to death. That is why I recommend multivitamin and mineral supplements and a nutritional checkup. The body utilizes the vitamins it needs and discards the excess. The requirements of the body for these vitamins will vary from day to day, however, depending on the foods taken in and the activity involved.

Naturally, the question arises about the use of large doses of vitamins so common today with health fadists. It is very well established now that large doses of Vitamin A and D can be very harmful. Definite, positive value from large doses of the other vitamins has not been established. I would recommend that you go easy on dosing yourself with vitamins until more is known, otherwise you could end up several years down the road being one of these unfortunate souls who find out too late that they've hit a *dead* end.

I once treated a young fellow of thirty-six in the hospital for a heart attack. Toward the end of his successful hospital stay he presented me with a book expounding the virtues of Vitamin E in preventing heart disease and commented, "Hey doc, you ought to read this. I've been taking Vitamin E for years." Obviously he didn't follow a healthy diet or life style to complement the vitamin E. The best advice that I can give at the present time is that if you *must* have a sense of security in regard to vitamins, take one good combination multiple vitamin-mineral tablet a day and remember, though a little bit may be good, too much can be harmful.

There are two classifications of vitamins. The *fat soluble vitamins,* Vitamins A, D, E, and K, dissolve only in fats or oils. They are absorbed through the intestine in the presence of fat and bile. If either of these two substances are lacking, or if there is disease present in the intestinal wall, then these vitamins may not be absorbed. Because they cannot be dissolved in water, they cannot be carried out of the body through urine. This accounts for the problems that arise with the overdoses of Vitamins A and D. Because they cannot be excreted by the kidneys, they can accumulate and become toxic. Vitamin C and the B complex vitamins are the *water soluble vitamins*. Vitamin B-1 deficiency, the cause of beri beri, and niacin deficiency, which is responsible for pellagra, are almost unheard of in the United States today. Scurvy (Vitamin C deficiency) is something you read about in history books.

B complex vitamins are found in whole wheat products, fresh meats, fish, green vegetables, liver, milk, and eggs. Although white flour has had the portion of the grain removed that contains most of the vitamins, minerals and fiber, some are replaced by the bread and cereal companies, thus giving the name to vitamin-enriched products. The roughage provided by whole grain products is unfortunately missing. The B complex vitamins are necessary for the utilization of carbohydrates. If, however, we take in large amounts of sugar and alcohol (which contain no vitamins), then deficiency states can develop. In some countries where the diets consist of mainly sugar cane and rum, lack adequate variety, and are low in meats and vegetables, you can expect to see some of the deficiency diseases I mentioned.

The B Complex Vitamins

Thiamine, Vitamin B-1. Necessary for proper function of enzyme systems of the body, heart and nerve tissue. Deficiency of thiamine can cause symptoms of irritability, fatigue, and constipation. Yeast and wheat germ are rich sources of thiamine, but it is also widely distributed in common foods, especially pork, ham, liver, lamb, beef, peas, asparagus, breads, and cereals.

Riboflavin, Vitamin B-2. Important in enzyme reactions, it is particularly essential for the release of cell energy and for tissue maintenance. Deficiency of riboflavin results in cracking and splitting of the lips and angles of the mouth (cheilosis), eye strain, headaches, and light sensitivity. Sources: dairy products, liver, tongue, pork, fowl, eggs, salmon, tuna, turnips, spinach, broccoli, asparagus, winter squash, prunes, strawberries, bread, and cereals.

Pyridoxine, Vitamin B-6. Active in the synthesis and metabolism of amino acids. Deficiency results in abnormalities of the nervous system and anemia. Should be taken as a supplement during pregnancy and when taking birth control pills. Sources: pork, lamb, veal, glandular meats, milk, eggs, vegetables, wheat germ, and bananas.

Pantothenic Acid. Associated with metabolism and synthesis of amino acids, hormones, fatty acids, and hemoglobin (in red blood cells). Sources: Availability widespread, esecially in eggs, liver, yeast, salmon, broccoli, peanuts, and bread.

Vitamin B-12. Though rarely ever needed, a shot of B-12 is the most asked-for injection in most doctors' offices next to penicillin. Pernicious anemia, a disease of the red blood cells, is brought about by an inability of the body to absorb this vitamin through the intestinal tract. The vitamin is also responsible for the maintenance of nervous tissue and pernicious anemia is associated with degeneration of the spinal cord. This vitamin is very plentiful. It can be stored by the body for several years. It is found in meats, fish, shell fish, milk, and eggs.

Other Vitamins

Folic Acid. This vitamin is usually found in green leafy vegetables. Only small amounts are needed and deficiency states are rare. It is essential for growth, blood formation, and amino acid syntheses.

Biotin. Deficiency occurs only when a large amount of egg white is ingested. It will then cause weakness, loss of appetite, depression, and anemia. It is important in fatty acid synthesis and is provided in our diets by liver, organ meats, mushrooms, and peanuts.

Vitamin C. This vitamin is found in fruits, particularly lemons, oranges, and grapefruits, vegetables, especially red and green peppers, broccoli, onions, cabbage, tomatoes, spinach, and watercress. Many claims have been made for Vitamin C and they are currently being investigated. So far, there has been no absolute confirmation for the miracle uses of this vitamin. Vitamin C plays a significant role in the formation of *collagen,* the protein substance responsible for cementing body cells together. It is also involved in amino acid metabolism and the absorption of iron. It appears to be of great benefit to the body under conditions of stress. I personally endorse larger doses of Vitamin C.

Vitamin A. This vitamin is found mostly in dairy products. A yellow-pigmented substance called carotene is found in many vegetables and this is converted by the body into Vitamin A. Some vegetarians who have gone overboard eating great quantities of carrots to obtain large amounts of "natural" Vitamin A have actually turned a yellow-orange color, which is protective. Vitamin A is also found in leafy vegetables, tomatoes, pimientos, potatoes, and liver. Vitamin A is utilized by the body to make "visual purple," a substance found in the retina of the eye. It enables us to see in dim light. A deficiency of Vitamin A causes night blindness. It plays other roles in vision and is important in maintaining the health of tissue membranes, particularly on the surface of the eye. Lack of adequate Vitamin A causes destructive changes in the mucous membrane lining the nose, throat, and sinuses. Overdosing yourself with Vitamin A can result in nausea and vomiting, baldness, dry skin, pain and swelling of the arms and legs. Current investigations are being carried out to establish the role of beta carotene (Vitamin A precursor) in combatting cancer.

Vitamin D. This vitamin is responsible for absorption of calcium and phosphorous and for depositing it in bone. It is obtained from dairy products and cod liver oil. It is responsible for the healthy growth of bone. It is also available to the body from the effect of sunlight on our skin. Deficiency of Vitamin D is rare today, but an excessive amount from overdosage can cause our bones to become brittle.

Vitamin E. This vitamin is found chiefly in the germ oil of nuts and grains, in leafy vegetables, milk and eggs, vegetable oils and liver, and in wheat germ. Deficiency of Vitamin E exists because of processing of foods such as white flour, grains, and oils. It received considerable attention when a deficiency occurred in infants who were fed a specific commercial milk substitute that was deficient in Vitamin E. Recent studies indicate that Vitamin E plays a role in maintaining the health and integrity of cell membranes. It helps prevent the breakdown of red blood cells and one form of anemia (rare in the United States). More about this later.

Vitamin K. Vitamin K, the "coagulation vitamin," is necessary for the maintenance of normal clotting of blood and also plays a role in metabolism of glucose. Deficiency of this vitamin is most likely to occur because of an inability of the intestines to absorb it rather than because of an inadequate supply in foods. Mineral oil and laxatives also interfere with its absorption. Excessive amounts of Vitamin A can be antagonistic to Vitamin K. It is found in many foods, including cabbage, spinach, cauliflower, leafy vegetables, vegetable oils, soybeans, and pork liver. It is poorly stored in the body and usually found only in the liver and in the linings of the respiratory, gastrointestinal, and genitourinary tracts. When deficiency occurs, protection against infection diminishes.

Vitamin and especially mineral deficiencies are very common in the United States. Recently, some vitamin deficiencies have appeared because of the use of new drugs in the armamentarium against disease. I have included a list of these so that you can quickly look through it, or show it to your doctor, to find out if you are on any of these medications and if, conceivably, it is causing the problem indicated. The subject of vitamin quackery will be covered in the chapter on "Magic, Myths, and Miracles."

MINERALS

There are many minerals which are required by the body for growth and the maintenance of good health. Careful research has indicated that it is very important that the body receive its requirements of minerals and that most individuals are deficient in one or more minerals due to dietary deficiencies.

Calcium. Calcium is readily available in dark green and root vegetables, cabbage, kale, almonds, kelp, soy and dairy products. It is utilized by the body for bone and tooth formation and in the process of blood coagulation. It plays a role in muscle contraction, including that of the heart. It is also used in many enzyme systems. The minimum requirement is 0.8 grams daily.

Phosphorous. In plentiful supply from salads, meats and poultry, fish, nuts, cheese, cereals, and legumes. Utilized in muscular and cell activity. The minimum daily requirement: 1.2 grams.

Iron. Available from meat, liver, legumes, whole grains, potatoes, egg yolks, dried fruits, and green vegetables. It is necessary for the formation of hemoglobin, the compound that carries oxygen in the blood. It is stored in the liver, spleen, and bone marrow. It is also utilized in the formation of myoglobin, which is the oxygen carrier in muscle tissue. Iron is also found in the enzyme system that brings oxygen to the cells. The minimum daily requirement: men, 10 milligrams (mg); women, 15 mg.

Iodine. Obtained in our diets from seafood, kelp, and iodized salt and in plants grown near the seacoasts. It is utilized by the body predominately in the formation of the thyroid hormone and, therefore, plays a major role in the rate of metabolism. The minimum daily requirement: .05–0.10 mg.

Sodium. Available in our diet predominately in table salt, in seafood, and in meats. It is extremely important in the mineral and water balance of the body. It is found in the extracellular fluid—that is, the fluids not contained within the cells but in the blood stream, around the cells, and in the urinary tract and gastrointestinal tract. The minimum daily requirement: .5 g.

Potassium. Available in meats, cereals, vegetables, and legumes. It is a component of the intracellular fluid—that is, the fluids within the cells. It plays a major role in the mineral and water balance of the body and in cell metabolism, particularly muscle metabolism, including the heart. The minimum daily requirement: 0.8–1.3 g.

Magnesium. Found in nuts, legumes, fish, corn, almonds, green and root vegetables. It is a component of bone tissue and is found in large amounts in muscle and blood cells. It plays a role in the enzyme metabolism of foods. The minimum daily requirement: 200–300 mg.

Chloride. Obtained in our diet mainly through table salt, seafood, and meats. Important in regulating the acid-base balance of the body, in the formation of hydrochloric acid in the stomach, and in regulating the mineral and water balance of the body. Daily requirement: .5 g.

Sulfur. Found in all tissues of the body. Part of the amino acid compounds and found in large amounts in hair and nails. It is available mostly in protein foods, especially eggs, and also in onions, garlic, cayenne pepper, meat, and fish.

Copper. Available in liver, nuts, and legumes. Important in the formation of hemoglobin and enzymes. Daily requirement: 2.0 mg.

Manganese. Available in bran, beets, peas, whole grains, blueberries, nuts, and vegetables. Daily requirement: Not established, but necessary.

Cobalt. Adequate amounts are usually present in our diet. Found in liver, leafy vegetables, fish, whole cereals. It is utilized in the body in the formation of red blood cells, is part of the structure of Vitamin B-12, and is essential to the nervous system. Excessive amounts of cobalt can cause an over-production of red blood cells.

Zinc. Zinc has been found to be utilized in the formation of body tissue and in the enzyme system regulating carbon dioxide metabolism. Recent studies have uncovered indications that zinc is important in wound healing, normal growth, and the metabolism of emotional behavior. Zinc in the body appears to exist in levels reciprocal to the levels of copper. In other words, an abundant intake of zinc may cause an excretion of excess copper and vice versa. Zinc deficiency may cause a loss of taste and smell. It may have some relationship to level of intellect. Current investigations with reference to zinc and copper in the immunological and allergic systems of the body are now going on. Sources are fish, kelp, peas, and lentils. The minimum daily requirement is not established, but is probably 20–30 mgs/day.

Water. We can function for long periods of time without food, but probably only several days without water. Between half and two-thirds of the body is composed of water. That includes cells (intracellular fluid) and all of the secretions of the body, the blood, and the lymph (extracellular fluid). It is the basic environment in which all of the reacions of the body take place. It regulates body temperature. It is the medium by which circulation, digestion, absorption, transportation, lubrication, and excretion take place. Water is supplied to the body mainly through the intake of fluids, although many foods contain water to a varying degree. Water is also produced in the body as an end product of metabolism. A deficiency of water causes a condition called dehydration, which can be fatal. It has been estimated that a twenty percent loss of body water can cause death. Next time you think of taking a diuretic (water pill) without a doctor's guidance, think of that. We will discuss water further under Metabolism (Scene 3). Daily *pure* water intake recommended is 1–2 quarts per day; more with vigorous physical activity and hot weather.

DRUGS AND THE DEFICIENCIES THEY CAUSE

Long-Term Therapy

Drug	Deficiency and Condition
Alcohol	Depletion of Vitamin C, folic acid, thiamine, riboflavin, niacin, Vitamins B-6 and B-12
Aluminum Hydroxide antacids	Osteomalacia due to phosphate depletion
Aminosalicylic acid (PAS)	Megaloblastic anemia related to Vitamin B-12 absorption
Anticonvulsants Phenytoin (Dilantin)	Depletion of Vitamin C due to malabsorption; calcium deficiency, rickets, and osteomalacia due to breakdown of Vitamin D
Ascorbic acid (megadoses)	Vitamin B-12 due to malabsorption
Calomel (HgCl)	Osteomalacia due to phosphate depletion
Cholestyramine resin (Questran)	Fatty stools, deficiencies of fat-soluble vitamins A, D, and K; iron deficiency, malabsorption of folic acid
Colchicine	Vitamin B-12 due to malabsorption

Long-Term Therapy (continued)

Contraceptives, oral	Vitamin C due to malabsorption, Vitamin B-6 due to increased urinary excretion
Cycloserine (Seromycin)	Pyridoxine depletion
Diuretics, all	Magnesium due to large doses and prolonged dosage
Diuretics, nonthiazides, such as furosemide (Lasix), ethacrynic acid (Edecrin), and triamterene (Dyrenium)	Calcium. Prolonged use and high doses could lead to decalcification and bone changes.
Ethionamide (Trecator)	Pyridoxine depletion
Hydralazine (Apresoline)	Polyneuritis due to antagonism of Vitamin B-6
Isoniazid	Convulsions due to pyridoxine depletion
Laxatives containing phenolphthalein or biscacodyl	Protein-losing bowel disease
Methotrexate	Megaloblastosis, anemia, and hepatic fibrosis due to folate antagonism
Mineral oil	Vitamins A, D, or K due to malabsorption
Neomycin sulfate	Fat, nitrogen, sodium, potassium, and calcium due to malabsorption
Penicillamine (Cuprimine)	Zinc due to malabsorption, pyridoxine depletion
Pentamidine isethionate (Lomidine)	Megaloblastosis and anemia; folate antagonism
Phenformin HCI (DBI, Meltrol)	Vitamin B-12 due to malabsorption
Phenytoin (Dilantin)	Folate antagonism
Potassium chloride, slow-release preparations (Kaon-Cl, Slow-K)	Vitamin B-12 due to malabsorption
Pyrazinamide	Pyridoxine depletion

Long-Term Therapy (continued)

Pyrimethamine (Daraprim)	Megaloblastosis and anemia; folate antagonism
Salicylates	Vitamin C due to malabsorption
Tetracyclines	Vitamin C due to malabsorption
Triamterene	Megaloblastosis and anemia; folate antagonism
Trimethoprim-sulfamethox-azole (Bactrim, Septra)	Megaloblastosis and anemia; folate antagonism

Scene 3
Metabolism—The Magnificent, Mystifying Machine

By nature, all men are alike, but by education become different. The essence of knowledge is to properly apply it; not having it, confess your ignorance.

Have you ever heard of the American Society of the Fist and Foot? As I understand it, Joe the Glut was one of the founders. If you watch the people around you carefully, you can usually pick out members of that Society by their unusual behavior. A normal day in Joe the Glut's life can provide you with typical examples of the Fist and Foot technique. Last Thursday, Joe the Glut got up at 5:00 A.M. to go fishing. He sat up at the edge of his bed and turned on the lamp on his night table. When it didn't go on, he took his fist and knocked the lamp off onto the floor. Somehow he had failed to notice that the lamp wasn't plugged into the wall. He went into the bathroom and got on the scale (you know about Joe and his scales). The dial wouldn't register so he kicked it across the room. He hadn't bothered to notice that the scale was half on the floor and half on the rug, and that the rug fibers were jamming the balance mechanism. When he finally got dressed and took all of his fishing equipment out to the car, his car wouldn't start. He turned the key; not a sound. Had he looked under the hood, he would have seen that the cable to the battery was disconnected. As he walked back to the house he kicked the right front tire, which promptly went flat. It is probably just as well that Joe didn't get to go fishing that day, because the last time he went fishing he became frustrated and angry over the fact that everyone else was catching fish and he wasn't (he had forgotten to bait his hook). He tried to put his fist into the mouth of the fellow who caught the most fish on the boat. The stranger was a karate expert in addition to being a good fisherman. Unfortunately, Joe found out that the Fist and Footers were no match for the Kamakazi Karate Kings of Kalamazoo.

The moral of the story is, of course, that you can avoid a lot of heartaches and possibly save a broken toe and a few front teeth by knowing how things work. And so it is with obesity; by knowing how your body works, losing weight becomes an enlightening and meaningful experience. The frustration that Joe the Glut felt came from his ignorance and was because he didn't bother to check things out. You can avoid frustration by gaining a greater understanding of what food is, what it is made of, what happens to food after you've eaten it, how it is processed by your body, and how it is converted into energy and fat.

METABOLISM

The food that we eat must be digested, absorbed, and used, and waste products must be excreted. This entire process is referred to as metabolism. It involves the breakdown of nutrients and their conversion into energy, which is referred to as catabolism. It also involves the manufacture and synthesis of new tissue and other products, and this is referred to as anabolism.

Carbohydrate Metabolism

When we take food into our mouth, it is crushed and chopped into smaller pieces and mixed with saliva, which contains an enzyme that begins the process of digestion. The enzyme, *amylase*, begins to digest starch in the mouth. The food is swallowed and enters the stomach where it is mixed with acid. The acid in the stomach stops the digestive action of amylase.

This brings up a profitable suggestion. In order to prolong the action of amylase, chew your food more thoroughly and keep it in contact with your tongue; you will not only taste it longer, but you will get the digestive process off to a better start.

The food goes from the stomach into the first part of the small intestine called the *duodenum*. There, intestinal juices are secreted and are again mixed with the food so that further digestion takes place. In addition to the enzymes secreted in the duodenum, hormones are released that send messages to other organs asking them for help. One of these organs, the *pancreas*, secretes enzymes and hormones into the intestine and bloodstream, assisting in the process of digestion. It is in the small intestine (of which the duodenum is the first part) that carbohydrates are broken down into the basic sugars—*glucose, fructose,* and *galactose.* These substances are absorbed through the wall of the small intestine and into the bloodstream. Practically all of the galactose and fructose are converted to glucose before absorption. Keep in mind, therefore, that *glucose is the basic form in which carbohydrates are absorbed into the body.*

This rather rapid absorption of almost all carbohydrates into the bloodstream in the form of glucose gives the physician the opportunity to check the metabolism of glucose, especially if diabetes is suspected, by testing blood glucose levels. In the most definitive test for diabetes, a five hour glucose tolerance test, the first blood sample is taken after the patient has fasted for fourteen hours. The patient is then given a measured amount of glucose to drink in the form of a specially prepared soda. Blood samples are then taken one-half, one, two, three, four, and five hours after drinking the soda. Urine samples are taken simultaneously with the blood samples. The level of blood sugar in each of these successive samples reflects the ability of the body to absorb glucose into the bloodstream and then remove it from circulation into the process of metabolism. The urine is also tested for traces of glucose.

The fuel for our brain is glucose. The rapid processing and absorption of glucose accounts for the fact that we can get a quick pick-me-up from a piece of candy or a drink of soda. With many individuals, mid-morning or mid-afternoon snacks perk up the thinking processes and provide a temporary boost in brain energy. When glucose is absorbed, it is carried in the bloodstream to the liver where *glycogen* is formed and may be stored as an energy reserve. Some glucose may be converted into fat (triglycerides), which is why you should limit sugar consumption, or into amino acids by the liver. The liver also completes the conversion of the absorbed sugars, fructose, and galactose into glucose. A little later on you will be shown how fat and amino acids can also be converted into glucose. Glucose is then delivered from the liver to the bloodstream and from there to the brain, muscles, and fat cells. The utilization of glucose by muscle depends upon the hormone *insulin* which is secreted from the pancreas. The level of glucose in the blood signals the pancreas to put out insulin. The higher the blood glucose, the more insulin is produced. In diabetes, this mechanism is faulty and an insufficient amount of insulin is produced, thus causing the blood glucose level to rise because it cannot be used by the muscle and fat cells. The kidneys act as a dam which holds back sugar from appearing in the urine. A very high level of blood glucose causes the sugar to spill over the dam into the urine. This provides many diabetics with a simple way to check the adequacy of their diet and medications in controlling their diabetes. If they are "spilling" sugar into their urine it is an indication that their blood sugar level is too high.

In muscle, glucose is stored as glycogen and is utilized to provide energy. However, most energy is stored in fat cells. Our muscles can also use fats and amino acids as a source of energy. Excess glucose is converted into fat for storage. Insulin plays a major role in the regulation of the transfer, storage, and conversion of glucose to fat. If your diet is not adequate in supplying glucose for these functions, then the body has to obtain it from the conversion of fatty acids and amino acids into glucose. This is important to remember later on when we discuss fad diets. When you've been conned into going on a low carbohydrate or no carbohydrate diet, your body, under rather stressful circumstances, must manufacture the glucose itself. Lopsided diets *produce* the problems, not relieve them. The fat cells store glucose by converting it into fat. In this situation, you can see that a low fat diet won't necessarily prevent obesity because glucose can take its place. The real answer lies in the total number of calories taken in, regardless of their source. The storage of large amounts of fat causes the fat cells to swell, and as we have already noted, obesity is caused by the increase in both the number and the size of the fat cells.

Cellulose is another carbohydrate that enters our body, but it is not digested because we do not have enzymes to do the job. It is the substance that makes up the fiber content of most vegetables. The main role of fiber is to provide bulk in our diet so that our digestive system can work more efficiently. Recently, great attention has been paid to the importance of the part that fiber plays as a possible bowel cancer preventative. It has long been known that fiber is a mechanical stimulant to the bowel promoting regularity of the bowel movements. Current research is investigating fiber's influence in stimulating the production and secretion of various substances which may play a role in protection and normalization of bowel function. To some degree, eating foods of high fiber content can prove to be rather filling without the body absorbing many calories.

Protein Metabolism

The digestion of protein begins in the stomach through the combined efforts of *hydrocholoric acid* and an enzyme called *pepsin*. Pepsin only works well when there is acid present. If you take too much antacid, especially while eating your meals, you will retard the digestion of protein. Aside from secreting digestive substances, the stomach also mixes up its contents by the contracting waves of the muscles in its walls. These are healthy movements and they are not usually felt like the painful spasms that you get when you have a stomachache. It is the presence of food itself that causes the flow of juices and the movement or contraction in the digestive tract. Proteins are also digested by duodenal, small intestine, and pancreatic juices. They are broken down into their component amino acids and absorbed into the bloodstream.

At this point, several things can happen to the amino acids. Some of them are transported to the liver where they are used to make plasma proteins. These are important ingredients in the composition of the blood. Other amino acids are converted by the liver into those amino acids that may be in short supply. The liver also removes nitrogen from the amino acids and converts the remaining product into glucose for energy, or into fatty acids for conversion into fat. It is important at this point to take special note of the fact that protein can be converted into glucose (carbohydrate) and fat. Here again, the ability of the body to perform this conversion casts doubt on the prudence of following absurd lopsided diets. Some of the amino acids are sent from the liver to the muscle, bone, brain, and in fact all of the tissues, including blood, that utilize amino acids for repair and replacement. Muscle and bone tissue, in particular, utilize most of the amino acids of the body. The tissue is being changed continuously, new tissue replacing the old. The used or worn-out amino acids are brought back to the liver for reprocessing. The buildup and breakdown of protein tissue may or may not be in balance. The processes of buildup or breakdown may predominate at alternating times depending upon what is going on in the body. When we are developing our muscles, for example during work or play, the buildup phase predominates. If, however, we were starving, the breakdown process would predominate. In the presence of an unbalanced diet, the lack of adequate amounts of glucose might cause the breakdown of protein and fats to provide fuel. It is important to note here that both fats and carbohydrates are necessary in our diet in order to spare our tissues from the breakdown of protein.

There are various glands that influence protein metabolism and the balance between construction and breakdown. Sex hormones, pituitary growth hormones, and insulin from the pancreas favor the buildup of tissue. Adrenal cortisol and thyroid hormone favor the breakdown of tissue. When the amino acids are broken down, nitrogen is removed and converted into urea (a waste product) by the liver. It is then excreted from the body in the urine. An increase in excretion of urea is indicative, then, of the fact that muscle is being broken down in excessive amounts. If there is any problem with kidney function, the excessive urea may accumulate and the condition called *uremia* may result. This could lead eventually to coma and death. Some individuals have been cautioned by their doctors about eating excessive amounts of protein in the form of meat, liver, and sweetbreads because of a condition called *gout*. These substances are high in purines, a breakdown product of certain proteins. Individuals with gout cannot process the *uric acid* which arises from the metabolism of purines. The uric acid crystallizes and may be deposited in the joints and the kidneys, causing arthritis and kidney stones. Both of these conditions can be extremely painful and interfere with the functions of and ultimately destroy joint and kidney tissue.

Fat Metabolism

The primary function of fat is that it acts as a means by which we store energy. You will recall that carbohydrates may be stored as glycogen for energy, but only in small amounts. Therefore, if we are to have a ready source of energy at all times without having to eat continuously, then there must be a way of storing it, and fat is that way. Because fat provides nine calories per gram, whereas protein and carbohydrates provide only four calories per gram, it is the most efficient form in which energy can be stored.

Fats are digested in the small intestine (the duodenum) and broken down into fatty acids. The process is assisted by the flow of bile from the liver and gall bladder, which breaks up the fat into small droplets. The pancreatic juices also play a major role in the digestion of fats. Neutral fat, fatty acids, and glycerol are then absorbed through the walls of the intestine into the bloodstream. After absorption, the fatty acids are converted back into fat by being combined with glycerol, which comes from the breakdown of glucose. The fat is transported to the liver, muscle, and fat storage cells by way of the lymph system and then the bloodstream. There is strong evidence that high fat content in the blood-stream leads to the formation of fatty plaques on the blood vessels, causing arteriosclerosis and heart disease. In the process of being transported, the fat droplets are either linked with or converted into albumen, cholesterol, and phosphates. In the presence of a sufficient supply of glucose for energy, most of the fat is stored in the fat deposits of the body. If there isn't enough glucose present, then the fat can be taken from the tissues, converted to glucose, and utilized by the muscle cells as a source of energy. Fat may also be removed from storage deposits to provide additional energy. If there is an overabundance of fats entering the body, the excess will be stored in the tissues. The breakdown from the processing of large amounts of fat produces excessive amounts of waste products called *ketones*. A portion of this substance can be utilized by the muscle of the body as long as adequate glucose is present. If the glucose is not present, even more ketones are produced and carried through the circulation to the kidneys, where they are excreted. If the kidneys cannot handle the excessively large amount, it piles up in the circulation and a condition called *ketosis* occurs. Obviously, therefore, glucose *must* be available in the body (carbohydrates *must* be present in the diet) so that ketones will not build up in the blood and cause ketosis. The body attempts to neutralize this condition with chemical substances called *bases*. Bases can be considered the opposite of acids, and it is the balance between these two substances that keeps the body chemistry neutral. Ketones are acid and combine with available bases, upsetting the chemical balance in such a way that other acid products of the body can predominate and a condition called *acidosis* occurs. At the same time, the kidneys try to flush out the excessive amounts of these waste products, and the loss of excessive fluid results in dehydration. These two conditions cause serious problems in body metabolism and can result in death.

The condition ketoacidosis occurs in severe cases of diabetes with the same consequences, even though the cause may be slightly different. In diabetes, the lack of insulin does not allow the muscle to use glucose. Fat is then broken down in an attempt to provide energy. Ketones are again produced and the body again tries to flush out the excessive glucose and ketones. Large amounts of body fluid are used in the flushing process. Excessive urination is a cardinal symptom of diabetes.

Glucagon and growth hormones cause the breakdown of fat. Insulin, on the other hand, tends to retard the breakdown of fat and in fact encourages its deposition in the tissues. In recent years there has been renewed interest in the problem of diabetes. A better understanding of the role of insulin, glucagon, and other substances should be forthcoming. It is to be hoped that studies will shed light on the role of these substances in causing obesity. Obese people have a forty percent higher incidence of abnormal carbohydrate metabolism. Their insulin level is usually increased. Abnormalities in the biochemistry of the body, usually found in obese individuals, can be caused in slender individuals by placing them on fattening diets.

The obese individual seems to have a problem with the storage of food surplus, which differs from storage processes in normal individuals. If an obese individual takes in 1000 calories consisting mostly of carbohydrates, that person's weight will increase by 50–100 grams in a twenty-four hour period. If the 1000 calories are taken in as fat, the individual will lose approximately 300–400 grams in twenty-four hours, and if the 1000 calories are taken in as protein, 100–200 grams will be lost during the twenty-four hour period. This does not mean that you can take in unlimited amounts of any of these substances and lose weight.

CHOLESTEROL

Cholesterol is a substance created in the body by the liver from protein, carbohydrates, and fat. It is also obtained from foods that we eat in our diet. The tremendous publicity given to cholesterol in recent years has created the impression that cholesterol is all bad. This is not true at all. Cholesterol forms bile in our bodies that is used for digestion, and is also used in the formation of Vitamin D. As with all of the substances I have discussed, it is either too little or too much that creates the problem. The cholesterol level in the body can be controlled by eating less saturated fat and more unsaturated fat, by cutting down on excessive food intake, and by engaging in more physical activity. However, the results of the latest research to reach the medical journals indicates that cholesterol control can be accomplished in select situations and to a limited degree. It appears that cholesterol metabolism is governed more by internal affairs than external contributions, and that the genetic makeup of the individual is of prime importance.

Food is more than just a source of fuel that provides our bodies with energy, energy that keeps the body itself working and energy that the body expends in doing work; it also supplies the materials for the body's construction, maintenance, and repair.

I think a little review of some of the salient points of the previous discussion on metabolism will help reinforce your understanding. The body's capabilities include the following:

1. It converts all absorbed sugars into glucose.
2. It can convert glucose into amino acids and fatty acids.
3. It can convert amino acids into glucose and fatty acids.
4. It can convert fatty acids into amino acids and glucose (all of the basic food substances can be converted from one form into another by the body).
5. It can convert one amino acid into another.
6. Insulin is necessary for muscle to utilize glucose.
7. When the body is not provided with adequate amounts of either carbohydrates, proteins, or fats, the deficiency will be corrected by the breakdown of various tissues and their conversion into the needed substances.
8. The breakdown of fatty acids creates ketone bodies.
9. The breakdown of protein creates urea.
10. Excess glucose is converted into fat for storage.

11. Most energy is stored in the body in fat cells.
12. Muscles can store energy in the form of glycogen.
13. Glucose must be present in order for muscle to utilize ketone bodies for energy.

Keep this list in mind and be ready to refer back to it when we discuss the fads and the fallacies of dieting. It should become obvious, even at this point, that a balanced diet containing carbohydrates, proteins, and fats is necessary in order to maintain a healthy body.

Some individuals have great difficulty in losing weight, even though they stick to a diet. Some of the theories and some evidence should be presented in an attempt to explain the physiological and biochemical problems that are involved in the problem of obesity. The basic concept that energy imbalance in intake and output is the essential cause of obesity still holds, but there are some modifying factors that keep it from being a simple matter of arithmetic. For example, one would think that a person who takes in three energy units in the form of food and burns up two would be left with one, which we have always assumed is stored as energy in the form of fat. We do know that there are two areas of the brain in the hypothalamic region that, when stimulated, will cause either eating or the cessation of eating. If these areas are destroyed, the opposite effects will occur, respectively. We also know that the intake of food is governed by levels of sugar in the blood, amino acids in the blood, the kind and amount of food eaten, the amount of bulk present in the stomach, and the general physical state of the body. With all of these known factors having an influence on the eating patterns of an individual, it is certainly not surprising that human beings differ in varying degrees from one another. However, other factors are also present that can stimulate a variation in food intake. Our fat cells, which are adapted for storing fatty acids as triglycerides, apparently rotate this fatty substance just as all the other tissues of the body are rotated. Triglycerides are formed from glucose and from lipoproteins under the action of hormones and enzymes. They are converted into fatty acids and glycerol by other hormones and enzymes. Insulin, epinephrine, glucagon, lipoprotein, lipase, prostaglandins, adrenal hormones, and thyroid hormones are just a few of the many substances involved in this very complicated process. It becomes very understandable that any minor variation, inefficiency, or deficiency in the functioning of this complicated process could result in the differences between human beings and their response to the amount of food that they eat. Bemoaning the fact that a friend of yours can eat as much as he or she wants to and still not gain weight simply will not do *you* any good. The reasons for the variations in storage of fat are not known, and even if they were known it would not mean that we could do anything about it, at least not right away. One interesting theory has it that the body behaves in this plentiful food supply society of today much as it did under primitive conditions when people had to store energy at times of feast to cover the times of famine. The fact remains, however, that we do not know the *reasons* and we do not have the *cures* for the differences in body type. The future will undoubtedly provide all of the answers, but that future may belong to our grandchildren and not to us. It makes more sense for us to say to ourselves, "This is the way it is now, this is what I have to deal with now. If I live in anticipation of the future, I lose the present." It is important for both the doctor and the patient to develop a greater acceptance and understanding of the difficulties and vexing questions that confront us in this problem and a tolerance of the metabolic differences that definitely exist among individuals attempting to lose weight.

It has been noted that a common factor in the eating habits of the obese is a tendency to overeat in the evening. Another study revealed that the obese individual exercises far less than the nonobese individual. In one particular study which compared the food intake and levels of activity of twenty-eight obese females and twenty-eight nonobese females, the obese girls ate less but also exercised less than the nonobese girls. It was also demonstrated that increased exercise does not increase food intake, and that therefore, exercise can be and is an effective weight control technique.

One of the issues that has plagued physicians for decades is the problem of some patients who swear that they have stuck to their diets and haven't lost weight. I can think of one sixteen-year-old girl in my practice who brought in her written list of food, totalled each day at 1000 calories, plus or minus fifty, who had gained one pound in a month's time. Her bowel habits had remained normal. She had not taken any excessive salt. Her diet, unfortunately, was not a balanced one. But even so, considering the fact that she was active in soccer and sports, she should have lost something. The only reasonable answer, at the current stage of medical knowledge, was that she must be holding fluid, in spite of the fact that she showed no outward evidence of this. I have read interesting theories about overtaxation of the enzymes and hormonal response in the bodies of obese patients causing them to produce fat even while following a low-calorie diet, but regardless of any enzyme or hormonal malfunction, body physiology should not be able to contradict the law of thermodynamics. If people are burning up more calories than they are taking in, they *must* be losing weight, or at least they *should* be. This is another reason why I recommend a balanced diet.

A balanced diet is one in which energy in the form of calories is provided for the body in the following proportions: Approximately twenty percent from protein, thirty percent from fats, and fifty percent from carbohydrates. These proportions were arrived at through careful investigations conducted in our most noted nutritional and medical research institutions. If your diet approximates these percentages, stresses on the metabolism of your body are less likely to occur. These are broad-based averages and may not apply to each individual.

The needs of the body have been spelled out for you and the reasons for these needs have also been explained. Let us take another step in increasing our knowledge by investigating the relationship between obesity and disease.

The plot thickens!

Scene 4
Obesity—Mother of Many Diseases

*Whatsoever was the father of disease, an ill diet
was the mother.*

It all began when Joe the Glut was a little boy. He must have been about two years old when his mother started to play the "I See You" game with him. That's the game where mommy puts her hands over her eyes, takes them away, and says, "I see you." Little Joe would mimic his mommy, doing the same thing, only he had the idea that when he put his hands over his eyes mommy couldn't see him either. A year or two later when he played the same game with mommy, he still felt that if he put his hands over his eyes, his mommy couldn't see him. Of course, mommy went along with it and reinforced this idea in Joe's little head. Now Joe was a smart kid. He figured that if it worked with his eyes, it would probably work with his ears, his mouth, his nose, and everything else, including his thinking. It seemed to work while Joe was a little boy, but when he grew up things started to catch up with him. He was hunting in the forest one misty morning. Another hunter aimed his gun at Joe, thinking that he was a wild animal (Joe did sometimes give that impression). Instead of running for cover, Joe put his hands over his eyes. It took them all afternoon down at the emergency room to get the buckshot out of his backside.

Maybe you're a proponent of the idea that "what you don't know won't hurt you." When it comes to your health, however, it's not a very good idea. Many patients have symptoms which frighten them, yet they avoid seeing the doctor for fear it will turn out to be something serious. It is *not* finding out that may be serious. Discovery and knowledge offer hope. Over the past twenty years I have discovered cancer of the cervix in women who hadn't had their cancer smears taken for several years. These women had been afraid to find out if something was wrong. Like children, they pulled the covers over their heads so that the goblins wouldn't get them. For some of these women, the price of fear and ignorance was their lives.

There is just no arguing with Mother Nature. We have learned to control her substantially in the last fifty years, but she is still in the driver's seat, especially when it comes to heart disease, cancer, and quite a few other problems in medicine. However, we—or rather you, the patient— can give her a good run for her money. Preventive medicine is really the patient's job. The doctor is only an adviser. The doctor will do everything possible to get you started, everything that's honest, sincere, and safe. The doctor won't lie to you and doesn't want you to lie to yourself. It's important to know as much as possible about the problems of obesity.

I'd like to give you a little background information about obesity and the diseases to which it is related or has some contributory effect. I want to scare you, scare you enough to shake you out of your complacency, scare you enough so that you will be able to sleep at night knowing that you've done *your* job. The word *doctor* means *teacher* and if I can teach you to enjoy your life, keep it healthy, and keep it long, then I will have done my job.

VASCULAR AND RELATED PROBLEMS (BLOOD VESSELS, HEART, AND KIDNEYS)

Obesity plays a significant role in the formation of a disease called *atherosclerosis,* which is a type of arteriosclerosis, or as it is commonly known, hardening of the arteries. Atherosclerosis predisposes people to coronary heart disease, abnormalities of the electrical functioning of the heart, and the formation of emboli or clots. Diabetes and hypertension are two other major diseases in which atherosclerosis plays an important role. The incidence of heart disease is markedly higher in patients who have either hypertension (high blood pressure) or diabetes, or both. The incidence of all of these conditions is greater in obese individuals, and all medical authorities agree that losing weight is an essential part of therapy. Another important fact is that all of the organs of the body rely upon circulation for healthy maintenance and function and will be adversely affected by the presence of atherosclerosis. The function of the kidneys in particular is markedly impaired by deficiencies in circulation. The kidneys are responsible for filtering waste products out of the blood and into the urine. If the filtering mechanism is not working properly, essential elements of the blood may be lost in the urine. In obese patients, particularly those with hypertension and diabetes, protein in the form of albumin is lost through the urine.

Obese individuals face a more serious complication arising from their hypertension. The dreaded cerebral vascular accident (stroke) occurs more frequently among the obese; it usually leaves a patient paralyzed and may result in death. Significant benefits are obtained by the majority of overweight patients when they lose weight. Blood pressure drops when as little as ten to fifteen pounds have been lost.

Because all tissue must be supplied by blood, the extra fat tissue requires the formation of extra blood vessels. This means that the heart has to do more work in order to supply these extra blood vessels with blood. If the rate of the heart remains unchanged, then the volume of blood pumped with each stroke must increase. As a result the left side of the heart, which provides the pumping force in the circulation, becomes enlarged and hypertension results. The rate may increase and place strain on the heart muscle.

Thus, obesity causes hypertension through two basic mechanisms. One is an increase in cardiac output or the amount of blood that the heart must pump, and the second is peripheral resistance or the blockage of blood flow. The increased resistance comes about through a combination of factors: increased body mass, stiffness and thickening of the vessel walls (atherosclerosis), and the release of toxins from the damaged kidneys. A vicious cycle of events occurs involving a complicated reaction in the body which eventually engulfs all major systems and organs and ends in disaster. To clarify your perception of the problem, let me give you a few statistics.

With obesity, the death rate from heart disease and kidney disease, primarily caused by blood vessel disease, is approximately fifty percent greater in men and seventy-five percent greater in women (than would be expected in the normal-weight population). Likelihood of cerebral hemorrhage or a stroke is about sixty percent greater than normally expected, and the likelihood of chronic kidney disease appears to be approximately one hundred percent greater.

For obese individuals who have had coronary attacks, the benefits of losing weight have now been well established. Weight loss even appears to reduce the pain of angina pectoris (the pain syndrome caused by lack of oxygen in the heart muscle).

Think about it; your heart has been beating day and night from a time several months before you were born until the present. Simple reasoning tells you that the heart is stronger and healthier when young. After it has been beating for several decades or more, why abuse it by carrying around extra fat? I am sure you have carried packages from the grocery store that weigh ten to twenty pounds for a distance of several blocks. How heavy they get; how uncomfortable you are! You sweat more, ache more, and breath more deeply. Look how you feel carrying only ten or twenty extra pounds. The stess of carrying ten to twenty pounds of extra fat is really not too different, although it's not as noticeable because the fat is more evenly distributed over your body. The older you get, the more important it is that you weigh what you did when you graduated from high school, or when you got married, or when you went into the service. *We should weigh less as we grow older, not more.*

Add to this another amazing fact: For every eight pounds that you are overweight, you carry a mile of blood vessels—that's 5,280 feet of extra blood vessels. True, most of these blood vessels are very small capillaries, but every inch of skin and fat must be supplied with blood. Your heart has to do the work of pumping the blood through these blood vessels. Is it fair to put a load on your heart after it has served you faithfully, twenty-four hours a day, for so many years? Consider, too, that the capacity and power of the pump remains relatively constant. When you add on those extra miles of blood vessels, you are diverting that power and flow of the pump from other areas. It stands to reason that you then deprive the vital tissues of your body, the vital organs, even the heart itself, of adequate blood flow and nourishment because you're siphoning it off to wasteful, unattractive fatty tissue. The vital organs are forced into a state of malnutrition and stress.

As a comparison, think of owning a home with a front lawn and a lawn in the back yard. You install a sprinkler system with a pump for the front yard and a pump for the back yard. The adequate irrigation or watering of your lawn keeps your lawn healthy and green. One day, however, the pump in your back yard burns out and you try to run the sprinkler system for both lawns off one pump. The one pump, of course, cannot handle the job adequately and the decrease in pressure causes brown rings to form on the lawn that is not receiving adequate moisture. The grass is dying of malnutrition and wilts at a faster rate. This is what is happening to the vital organs and tissues of an obese individual. They are dying at a faster rate. No wonder the insurance companies are reluctant to insure the obese. It also explains why the statistics associated with obesity are so depressing and why medicine currently views it as the greatest medical problem. In reality, it is the number one killer yet escapes being listed as such because it is a "condition" and not a "disease." The label is obviously unimportant. When your life is in danger, the classification of the threat provides little solace.

In general, excessive weight acts as a barrier to blood flow, particularly when a patient is in a standing position. The flow of blood back to the heart is encouraged by muscle contraction and is discouraged by compression. This is one of the reasons why doctors try to dissuade patients from wearing garters or constricting garments. Obese individuals are far more prone to developing *varicose veins* and *ischemic ulcers* (breakdown of skin due to a lack of adequate circulation). Because of the poor circulation they will very often complain of pain while walking, a condition called *intermittent claudication*.

The condition of *phlebothrombosis* is far more common in obese patients than in the normal population. This is a condition in which a clot forms in the veins of the body. If, for example, these clots or thrombi should occur in the renal veins, the functioning of the kidneys would be impaired and a condition known as nephrotic syndrome would be likely to occur. The connection is so striking that when the nephrotic syndrome occurs in an obese patient, it is advised that the physician search for a renal vein thrombosis. Heat stroke is also more common in obese individuals. The extra demand placed upon the circulatory system because of heat stroke can mean the difference between survival and death when a patient is obese.

RESPIRATORY DISEASE

The act of breathing is accomplished by muscle action in the chest wall and the rib cage. When additional weight is carried on the chest wall, the effort required to breathe is increased. There is less movement in the chest wall of an obese individual, and the exchange of oxygen and carbon dioxide is correspondingly less. With the retention of carbon dioxide, the patient has a tendency to become sleepy and less active. With a decrease in oxygen intake, there is a decrease in the transfer of oxygen to the blood and the diffusion of oxygen into the tissues of the body is diminished. The tissues of your body are forced to function under great stress. They are being suffocated and are dying at a faster rate. Obesity imposes another stress on the lungs by requiring the lungs to supply a greater amount of oxygen to a greater mass of tissue. This in turn poses or creates another problem. If oxygen is diverted to the excess tissue, then less oxygen is available for exercise or body movement. The tolerance for exercise diminishes and a destructive cycle comes into effect. A decrease in activity leads to greater obesity. This in turn leads to further decreases in activity. If a respiratory infection occurs, its effect on the obese individual is exaggerated. The body's defenses cannot be mobilized efficiently. Nothing seems to work as well and the risk climbs.

With inadequate ventilation and oxygenation, carbon dioxide tends to accumulate in the blood. The lack of adequate oxygen stimulates the blood-forming organs to produce excessive numbers of red blood cells. Red blood cells carry oxygen, and by multiplying them the body is attempting to compensate by raising its oxygen-carrying capacity in order to reach the tissues of the body. This increased number of red blood cells is called *polycythemia* and may lead to the formation of clots (thrombosis) and problems with clotting of the blood. The heart also becomes involved in this respiratory cycle; it attempts to make up for the lack of adequate oxygen in the blood by trying to pump harder. Consequently, the heart enlarges and failure of the heart muscles may occur. This is called congestive heart failure. As the heart fails to pump the blood into the general circulation, it backs up into the lungs, causing fluid literally to drown the lung tissue and block oxygen transfer. If unchecked, it eventually causes death. You can see that the effect of obesity on just one function of the body, breathing, can cause an infinite number of serious problems. Reflect for a moment before we look into other problems related to obesity. What I have discussed so far is already happening to you. The effect may be so slight that you are unaware of it, but it is happening. When the symptoms become obvious, the damage may be beyond adequate repair. Disease can be like a pot of water on a stove. Below 100° C, a hot or cold pot of water looks the same, but when it hits 100° it boils over. However, if you put your finger in the water at 99°, you burn your finger just as easily as when the water is boiling.

ARTHRITIS

There is no question that diseases of the joints and bone are more common and more severe in the obese individual. *Herniated (ruptured) disc disease* of the spine and *arthritis* are two major painful diseases that are not only worsened by obesity, but can be relieved considerably by losing weight. Arthritis is not a single disease entity but rather a term that is applied in a general sense to a whole host of diseases that affect the joints.

Arthritis can be caused by infection, and that technically means that any one of the known bacteria can cause infection in the joints. This kind of arthritis would be referred to as *infectious arthritis*. Let us say, for example, that you were out weeding your lawn and got a small piece of glass stuck in your knee. You neglected it and it became infected. That infection spread into the capsule of the joint. You would most probably get a staphylococcal infection, which would be called staphylococcal arthritis if the joint infection progressed to a point where the cartilaginous surface was eroded. In essence, the process of erosion of the cartilaginous surface and then of the bone is what occurs in all forms of arthritis, although the cause may be different in each case. Even gonorrhea has been known to cause arthritis, a little-known complication of this well-known venereal disease.

Arthritis can be caused by trauma or injury. The injury could be acute, causing, for example, the kind of arthritis that football players so frequently get in the knees. The injury could be chronic in nature, caused by the gradual wear and tear from normal use of the joints. This arthritis is referred to as osteoarthritis and is the most common form. Almost every human being will have it to some degree while aging. Rheumatoid arthritis, a particularly crippling form of arthritis, is believed to be caused by some derangement of the immunological system of the body, but its exact cause is not known. Arthritis can also be caused by a derangement of the metabolism of the body. In gout, for example, crystals of uric acid are deposited in the joint, causing erosion and inflammation of the joint structure.

A joint is the articulating surface where two bones meet and where movement takes place. They are held together by ligaments and muscles and their tendons. This should help you understand how excessive weight can complicate the disease process involved in arthritis. The hip joints and the knee joints are most frequently affected by excessive weight. These joints carry all of the weight above them when in the standing position. For example, if an individual weighed 250 pounds, approximately 210 pounds of that weight would be resting on the knees while that individual remained standing. With each step a person takes, too, the surfaces of the two bones of the knee grind together under great compression and weight. The erosion begun by the arthritic process, regardless of the cause, is seriously aggravated by the continued grinding under pressure of excess weight. This wear and tear creates an inflammatory process and heat, redness, and pain result. It is not unusual for a physician to see in his office, many times a year, individuals who are severely crippled and incapable of walking because of the marked destruction of knee joints. These patients are invariably overweight. The loss of weight does not cure the arthritis, but it reduces the friction and stress on the arthritic joints and relieves the pain considerably.

DIABETES

The type of diabetes that occurs in adulthood (maturity-onset diabetes) is dramatically affected by a loss in weight. In one study, seventy-five percent of those obese diabetics who achieved a normal weight achieved normal blood sugar levels at the same time. In diabetes, it is believed, the lack of insulin or some deficiency in its function does not allow for the proper utilization of glucose by the cells. The glucose is not available for metabolizing ketones in muscle tissue. Fat is then metabolized to compensate for the inability to utilize glucose, and a destructive cycle resulting in acidosis and ketosis results.

In diabetes, the loss of weight can help many patients avoid the need for taking insulin. It can lessen many of the complications of diabetes, particularly skin disease, infections, and the serious threat of diabetic acidosis. Until the cause or causes of diabetes are better understood and its cure is discovered, loss of weight and intelligent eating are the two most effective measures for combating its serious consequences.

GALLBLADDER DISEASE

The association between obesity and gallbladder disease is very striking. There is no evidence that by losing weight you necessarily correct a gallbladder condition, but if you lose weight and do not have a gallbladder condition, there certainly is less likelihood that you will get one. If you do have a gallbladder condition, at least your risk of surgery will be greatly lessened if you bring your weight down to normal. If an operation becomes necessary, then losing weight will reduce the risk of complications and even death at the time of surgery. This, of course, applies to all surgical procedures. I still remember from many years ago the advice of a professor in medical school, who instructed us always to look for gallbladder disease in patients who were fair, fat, and forty.

DIAPHRAGMATIC HERNIA

Diaphragmatic hernia (hiatus hernia) occurs more frequently among the obese. For those of you who are not familiar with diaphragmatic hernia, let me describe it for you. Your swallowing tube (esophagus) descends from your throat down through your chest and then through a hole in the diaphragm (that is, the sheet of tissue inside your body at the base of the ribs separating your lungs from your intestines). As soon as the esophagus passes through an opening in the diaphragm, it becomes the stomach. Now, if that opening in the diaphragm enlarges, then the stomach has a tendency to push up into the chest. This is called a diaphragmatic or hiatus hernia. It can be quite painful and cause severe symptoms of indigestion. Diaphragmatic hernias typically give patients more trouble when they are lying down than when they are standing up, when they eat large meals, and when they bend over at the waist. The weight of the intestines pressing against the stomach pushes it up through the diaphragm. In obese individuals, this weight and pressure is very great.

CANCER

Recent studies indicate that there is an increased risk of breast and endometrial cancer (cancer of the inner lining of the uterus) in obese individuals. The risk of endometrial cancer appears to be two to four times greater, especially in women who have been obese since their teen years, than among women of normal weight. The risk of breast cancer appears to be two and one-half times greater. It is believed that the excess estrogen found in obese post-menopausal women may be a major factor, another good reason for older women, in fact, all women, to bring their weight under control.

Cancer of the liver and gallbladder is 70 percent more frequent in men and 110 percent more frequent in women than it would be among their normal-weight counterparts. Incidence of cancer of the intestines and rectum is fifteen percent higher. The risk of cancer of the female organs, the uterus in particular, is twenty percent higher.

Statistical analyses of the incidence of various medical problems that occur in the obese population as compared to the normal population reveals some very startling comparisons. The following facts have appeared in responsible medical journals:

Incidence of diabetes is 300 percent greater
Cirrhosis of the liver 150 percent
Appendicitis 120 percent
Hernia and intestinal obstruction 50 percent
Gallbladder disease 50 percent
Gallstones 100 percent
Automobile accidents and falls 30 percent
Complication of pregnancy 60 percent
Cancer of the pancreas 50 percent greater in women

SKIN PROBLEMS

Obese individuals generally sweat more than normal individuals. The excessive perspiration and the heat and darkness created by the folds of excessive fat tissue provide an ideal culture environment for bacteria and fungus. Consequently, obese individuals have a greater incidence of fungal and bacterial rashes, inflammation, and boils.

CHILDBIRTH AND REPRODUCTION

Toxemia, a disease involving high blood pressure, edema (water retention), and kidney failure, is a serious problem in pregnancy and occurs much more frequently in the obese female. This condition can result in the death of the mother and the baby. The overweight woman may have more difficulty becoming pregnant, and is more likely to have problems with delivery.

The higher incidence of infertility in obese men may possibly be caused by the increased temperature in the area of the testicles because of the excessive weight.

Excess hair growth (hirsutism) and irregular menstrual cycles can often be changed for the better when obese women have lost weight.

Anemia, due to iron deficiency, occurs more frequently among obese subjects than it does in the general population.

THE PSYCHOLOGICAL EFFECTS OF OBESITY

In later chapters I will be discussing the emotional causes of obesity and the use of intellect and emotions in dealing with the problem of obesity, but it would be appropriate in this chapter on diseases to discuss the effects of obesity on an individual's feelings and life style. In other words, emotional problems may cause obesity, but obesity invariably causes emotional problems.

My wife and I recently made a trip to the Canadian Northwest. We travelled with about twenty other people in a beautiful, air-conditioned bus that had the marvelous convenience of a bathroom on board. One evening at dinner, one of the other passengers commented that a friend of hers would not have been able to make the trip. When her husband asked who that was, she said, "Jane, of course. With her weight and size, I don't know how she could even get through the door of the bathroom on the bus." This conversation made me stop and think about all the everyday activities that a fat person is prevented from doing.

Great strides have been made by society in providing special facilities for the handicapped. Attention has been paid to the crippled, the blind, and the deaf. Nothing has been done for the obese, yet the obese form the largest group of handicapped persons. Society does not look at the obese individual in the same way that it considers the traditional handicaps. In fact, obesity is not considered a handicap. Our society looks upon the obese as irresponsible, lacking in self-control, self-indulgent, and immature. They are considered to have a condition not brought upon them by the fates, but by themselves. Furthermore, obese people are victimized by their obesity. Aside from facing everyday physical limitations, they may become social outcasts and for the most part withdraw into a solitary existence. If hatred of self didn't cause the obesity, it eventually becomes a product of it. If obese children don't exclude themselves from the games other children are playing, the other children will often do it for them. If their self-image isn't impaired to begin with, their constant failure at dieting is sure to do it. They avoid looking in the mirror because they see themselves as repulsive and ugly. They can become sexually frustrated and emotionally deprived, as well as physically handicapped. They wear the brand of failure too conspicuously. The despair and rejection they feel from themselves and society leaves them little else to do but look for some small pleasure, some small comfort, some sweet taste in a bitter world. Where there is no love, food becomes love. When there is no one to console, food consoles. When life is without sex, food becomes sex. When life is without pleasure, food becomes pleasure, and if food is practically the only source of the sweet taste in a bitter world then the person gets fatter. But it needn't be so.

ACT 2
IN SEARCH OF THE TRUTH

How do I diet?
Let me count the ways.

Scene 1
Magic, Myths, and Miracles

Americans are an incredible people. They have incredible ideas, incredible energies, incredible wealth and power, and, oh yes, an incredible need to believe in miracles because of their incredible achievements. This, of course, makes them incredibly gullible.

One day, while touring our great western outdoors, Joe the Glut stopped off for a beer at a quaint little old western-style saloon. The sun was going down and an eerie haze hung over the land as dusk descended. Joe walked up to the bar and asked the burly bartender for a beer. The bartender peered at Joe with deep-set, dark, mysterious eyes. Without a sound or change in expression, he reached around, grabbed a bottle of beer, opened it for Joe and handed it to him. The floor boards creaked beneath Joe's feet as he walked back to a table and sat down. The bar room was dimly lit, and as far as Joe could tell there was nobody else in the room. He suddenly felt a chill going up the skin of his back and felt an uneasy foreboding. Just then, there was a rush of wind that caused a rattling sound at the window. The air seemed to cry and moan in sympathy with his frightened feelings. The door suddenly blew open and a strange man, dressed in tattered old prospector's clothes, appeared in the doorway. It seemed as though he had just landed in a chariot of swirling dust. The old man peered straight ahead at the bartender, who nodded his head in Joe's direction. The old man turned to look, closed the door behind him, and slowly moved toward Joe. Joe's fear became intense; he felt paralyzed and stuck to his seat. The old man, sensing his fear, said in a warm, calming voice, "Don't be startled, my son." Joe was now convinced that something strange was happening to him, that some great, mysterious event was about to take place. The reassuring voice immediately substituted trust for fear and tranquility for turmoil. Joe was spellbound!

The old man sat down at his table and started to unfold to Joe an incredible tale. He told of his thirty years of wandering as a man of nature, a man in search of ancient Indian medical cures. He spoke of mountain caves and secret places, of clandestine meetings with the witch doctors of various tribes. He recalled the hunger and starvation, the winter blizzards, the scorching summer's heat, and the countless lonely days. He described the moments of doubt, the feelings of frustration and failure. Joe was caught up in every word. He became totally involved in the adventure. His excitement grew as the search neared its end, his eyes filled with tears at the telling of the moment of victory. The old man described that moment with such emotion that Joe could swear that he heard organ music from the heavens and could see an aura of brilliant whiteness surrounding the old man's body. At last he had found his dream, the object of his quest, the great magical substance which was the essence of life, which made all things grow, the basic food of living cells, the core of nourishment, the fundamental substance.

The old man paused, nearing the end of his tale. His eyes cast downward, he spoke again, quietly and with great sadness, "My discovery has come too late and I am dying. I am old and I am tired. I wish to return to my home, touch the soil which gave birth to me, and breathe my last breath. All I need is my bus fare back to my beloved Virginia and a few dollars for food to nourish my tired body. For $100 I will give you my secret, the product of my life's work." He reached under his cloak and brought forth a large, irregular package wrapped thickly in brown paper. It was tied with many turns of rope and knotted very securely. Joe the Glut was deeply touched by the triumphant, yet tragic story. He reached for his wallet, took out five twenties, and handed them to the old gentleman. Joe gazed down at the package on the table, and by the time he again looked up, the old man had disappeared. Joe hastily put a dollar on the table, picked up the package, and ran to his car. His body trembled with excitement.

He drove for perhaps an hour until he found an out-of-the-way motel. Parking the car, he got out and looked around to make sure that no one was observing him. He went into the office and made arrangements for a room for the night. On the way to his room, he glanced over his shoulder again to make sure that he wasn't being followed. Once inside his room, he locked the door behind him and placed the package on the bed. His hands were shaking as he tried to wrestle with the thick cord, which it took him a full ten minutes to undo. Then he ripped off several wrappings of paper, several wrappings of waxed paper, and then several wrappings of plastic-wrap. As he gazed at his prize, his forehead broke out into beads of sweat. The blood rushed to his face and his heart pounded rapidly. For there, lying on the bed in front of him, was the essence of life, the essence of all growing things, the nourishing food for all cells, his fountain of youth, his unreachable star—a pile of horse-manure!

Charlatans and quacks have been around for a long time. Quacks of all sorts have claimed to cure people by radio waves, electrical waves, magnetic waves, thought waves, and an assortment of unheard-of waves that were unheard of and never heard of again. All kinds of gadgets have been sold, leased, and franchised; boxes to sit on, boxes to sit in, boxes to sit under, rings for your fingers, bracelets for your wrists, and collars for your neck made of copper, brass, hair from horsetails, and tails from asses. Mysterious undetectable beams have been bounced on people, off people, in people, through people, and back at people. The miracle merchants sold pills, tonics, nostrums, brews, garments, and you-name-its to millions of people for millions of dollars. Some of the great fakers even had streets, boulevards, and buildings named after them.

The list of worthless miracle materials continues to grow while the miracles never materialize. In the past twelve years, two "cancer cures" have caused widespread controversy and even involved disputes between state and national governments. One of them, Krebiozen, attracted the support of several respected medical investigators but proved to be adulterated mineral oil. The story of Laetrile is also entering its final chapter, and it appears that it too will fade into oblivion, leaving behind it a trail of dashed hopes and despair.

The perpetrators of these frauds invariably use testimonials to support their claims. You will never find carefully documented and controlled studies. Look through almost any magazine on the stands today and you will see advertisements for all sorts of medicines and gadgets for which testimonials are the only "proof." There will always be some people willing to give a testimonial that Preparation "X" cured them. In almost every instance, it is an unsubstantiated illness cured by an unsubstantiated drug. Frequently, unfortunate individuals who are suffering from terminal illnesses are subjected to the most unspeakable kinds of fraud. They are robbed of their funds, their dignity, their hope, and a chance for legitimate therapy. Actually, I can't blame the public too much for jumping on every fad bandwagon that comes along. A large amount of new knowledge is being discovered by the scientific community at a rapid rate. Most of this knowledge is published only in medical and scientific journals. Much of it can only be understood by highly-trained, specialized individuals. It may take many years before the significance of new discoveries can be fully comprehended and their role in our everyday lives determined. The public becomes confused and frustrated when new information reaches the media. Often it appears to be contradictory and at times may challenge well-established concepts. Laws and safeguards may be thoughtlessly discarded because public pressure and impatience may force the premature disclosure and application of new information before its impact on our way of life is fully and correctly interpreted.

In the field of nutrition and dieting, the food faddists get the most publicity. They achieve their fame through their ability to attract public notice. The statements made by most faddists are unfounded, designed to startle, attract attention, and make big profits. They start out with a small truth, which they exaggerate into a big lie. Their claims are baseless and backed by testimonials that are in turn backed by coincidence, imagination, and fantasy.

One of the quack axioms is "If a little is good, a lot is better." In reality, the opposite is almost always true. They usually start out with a truthful statement, add a "therefore," and end up with a conclusion that suits their needs, not yours. They deal in extremes and distortion. Another axiom frequently used is "If a lot of something is bad, then don't take any, or eliminate it completely," or, "If it is bad for one, then it is bad for all." Some quacks have said this about meats, others have said it about sugar, others about one vegetable or another, the water we drink, and the fruits we eat. If we took all of their advice together, we would have to stop eating. The one rule that everybody *should* follow is that "Too much of almost anything *can* be bad. Maturity mandates moderation." The very sad, tragic, and criminal result arising from the preachings of the faddists is that an individual may fail to obtain legitimate medical help in time.

Why do people follow the fads? I believe that some people feel the need to remain like children in some corner of their personalities. They want to believe in miracles, to believe that wishing makes it so, that dreams come true. For some, the fad promises something for nothing; for others, it is an opportunity to avoid the responsibility and the effort required to achieve a goal.

Very few aspects of living have attracted the merchants of magic, myths, and miracles as much as nutrition and dieting. When a particular diet is the "current rage," it arouses serious interest and enthusiasm on the part of the fat or potentially fat population. Everybody wants to try it, everybody wants their problem to disappear—pooff!

As I reviewed the history of dieting, I found diet references dating back to the ancient Egyptians, Greeks, and Romans. Advancement in the art of communication and the advent of the "best seller list" has since brought us an overwhelming number of books on diets for the obese. As I looked back over the era I had lived through, my opinion of these diets changed and I began to chuckle. I found them amusing, yet sad, like comedy that rises from the ashes of tragedy.

FAD DIETS—AN OVERVIEW

Any diet that advocates elimination of any one of the basic food substances, carbohydrates, proteins, or fats, seriously endangers an individual's health. Anyone who says that calories don't count defies a basic law in physics and simply demonstrates ignorance. Any diet claiming that you can take in as much of any of these three basic substances that you want and still lose weight is completely false. Eliminating fat from your diet simply means that the body will convert carbohydrates and proteins into fat instead. The same principle applies to proteins and carbohydrates, except that in the case of proteins, a deficiency of the essential amino acids will have serious consequences. All of these substances contain calories, and excess amounts of carbohydrates, proteins, or fat will be stored as fat in the body. Calories cannot be made to simply vanish. They must be either utilized (burned up) or stored. All of the notorious faddists and quacks of our day focus their attention on one or two elements of the process of metabolism. They would have you believe that one or two processes could be the sole determining factors in the utilization and disposal of energy. They totally ignore all of the complex processes we have reviewed and the serious consequences that can result from significant imbalances in the body's metabolic picture.

Let's take a closer look at some of the more popular rip-offs.

High Protein, High Fat, Low Carbohydrate Diets (Ketogenic Diets)

Predominately high protein diets include several limited and varying proportions of fat and carbohydrates. The possible consequences of these diets as cited by the National Board of Nutrition are ketosis, acidosis, hyperurecemia, hypercholesterolemia, fatigue, nausea, cardiac arrhythmia, hypotension, and disturbances of menstrual and ovulatory patterns.

Diets based on the concept that calories don't count have attempted to defy the law of thermodynamics and scientific fact established by biochemists, physiologists, nutritionists, and physicians all over the world— a very unique and brave stand, especially in view of the fact that the claims could not be substantiated (*Patient Care*, June 1, 1976, p. 83.) To add injury to insult, these diets are usually deficient in vitamins and minerals and are just variations of the old high protein, high fat, low carbohydrate diets. These are often referred to as the ketogenic diets, in which the effect of ketosis suppresses the appetite. It is the loss of appetite and thus a reduction in caloric intake that is responsible for the weight loss. Therefore, *calories do count.*

A theory was presented that excess weight is caused by the body's inability to metabolize carbohydrates properly. It suggests that patients restrict carbohydrates and increase the intake of protein and fat. It is claimed that weight loss results from a transformation of calories into ketone bodies which are lost in the urine. There is only one problem: this theory is completely unfounded scientifically. Biochemists state that it is almost impossible to lose more than 100 calories a day in ketones. As you already know, every gram of protein contains four calories and every gram of fat contains nine. If you're going to eat a lot of fat and protein, that's a lot of calories.

It is interesting that one author admits that his diet is similar to many of the other ketogenic diets. He did cite one difference, however, criticizing another author for the fact that he prescribed six glasses of water a day in his diet. Now that's a monumental difference! (*Medical World News,* April 27, 1973, p. 38.) Since you have learned about metabolism, how does it strike you that some diets ask you to develop ketosis? These diets are based upon eliminating carbohydrates from your diet until ketosis develops. One diet is loaded with saturated fats and cholesterol-rich foods, which as you educated readers already know are not desirable.

In addition to the problems cited above, the ketogenic diets cause a multitude of symptoms and side reactions: loss of calcium, dehydration (loss of body fluid), intolerance to exercise and exertion, elevated blood lipids and uric acid (watch out for atherosclerosis and gout!), and kidney stress, which is potentially dangerous to patients with kidney disease, and which may damage the gallbladder if the diet is followed during pregnancy. Unfortunately, the long-term effects of ketosis are not fully known at the present time. Without carefully monitored studies, the kind of fiasco that these diets could cause might go unrecognized for a considerable time, leaving a wake of irreparable damage behind it.

One author covered himself on both sides. In one diet, he prohibited the intake of seafood, poultry, meats, milk, and cheese. In the other diet, *he allowed an unlimited intake of these very same foods!* (*Patient Care,* June 1, 1976, p. 83.)

No matter what you name them, the net results of these diets are the same. The risks are high, the weight loss temporary, and you've learned nothing except how to unbalance your diet. The tab, the time, and the torture—all for nothing.

The Drinking Man's Diet is just another variation of the high protein, low carbohydrate diet. The risks here, in addition to those we have already discussed, are alcoholism and a more rapid downfall nutritionally. Alcohol is a significant cause of disease when its proportion of the total body intake of energy rises above fifteen to twenty percent. For example, if your total caloric intake is 2500 calories and 500 of those calories come from alcohol, damage to your tissues will take place regardless of how balanced or how good the rest of the diet might be. If the diet is unbalanced, the risks are even greater.

When the fat content in this group of diets is pushed excessively high, additional problems occur. A high fat diet depletes calcium from the system, increasing the risk of osteoporosis in post-menopausal women. This is in addition to the problems of elevated cholesterol and lipid levels discussed in the chapter on disease. The restriction of carbohydrates in these diets may deprive the brain and even the retina of the eye of adequate nourishment.

During pregnancy, low carbohydrate diets may be extremely hazardous because lactose and dextrose are essential for fetal brain development. Dizziness, fatigue, slowness and confusion of thinking processes, and difficulty of vision are not uncommon consequences of these diets. Whereas high protein advocates say that high carbohydrates make you fat, I would like to call your attention to the fact that vegetarians eat mostly carbohydrates and most of them are *not* fat. Remember the lesson from the chapter on metabolism? It is fat that we want to get rid of, and glucose (carbohydrate) is essential in the metabolism of fat. *Remember always that a balanced diet is your best protection against disease.* If, for example, you lower your fat intake while on a high protein diet, it may result in skin diseases, particularly eczema, and in liver malfunction. In addition, the balance of the flow and utilization of energy and of the constant repair and replacement of tissue will be hindered.

It is incredible that any physician would try to assert that the high protein diet is new or revolutionary, or to use any other adjectives to indicate that it is a recent discovery. The records show that Dr. William Banting, the British physician, introduced a high protein diet in 1864. The diet is essentially the same; only the names have changed. It is even more incredible that a physician would recommend an unbalanced diet to his patients. I am appalled by physicians who say "It's O.K." for you to go into a state of ketosis as long as they are watching you. The excuse given very often is that the "disease is still worse than the cure." How many of the patients that have gone on these ketogenic diets are in such a morbid state that they warrant such methods? Remember, the risks are high, the weight loss temporary, and the patient learns nothing except an unbalanced diet. The tab, the time, and the torture—all for nothing!

Starvation

Total starvation resembles the high protein, high fat, low carbohydrate diet. When food is withheld, the body feeds on itself. Starvation causes a loss of fifty to sixty-five grams of body protein a day for the first one to two weeks, a twenty-five to forty gram loss of protein each day after the second week, tapering down to fifteen to twenty-five grams of protein a day after that. The amount, of course, will be proportional to the size of the individual. Calcium and phosphorus are metabolized from skeletal tissue, causing the bone to become brittle and weak. Other effects of fasting are a reduced metabolic rate, negative nitrogen balance, ketosis, hypotension, cardiac arrhythmia, atrophy of the intestinal mucosa (lining), anemia, edema, nausea, weakness, apathy, lack of libido (decreased sexual desire), emotional and behavioral upset, and finally, disappointment and self-deception.

Crash diets or starvation diets usually cause approximately two-thirds of the weight loss to occur in muscle, liver, kidneys, and other vital organs of the body. These tissues require fatty acids and glucose as a source of energy. Without this source available, the body breaks down protein tissue along with the fat in order to continue functioning. Do you still want to fast? O.K. Mahatma, have it your way!

Starvation in Athletes

When an athlete starves himself prior to activity, he depletes the protein stored in the body and attacks the "lean tissues" such as the liver, pancreas, small intestine, and muscle. Consequently, the weight is being lost from areas that can ill afford it. This is in addition to the problems of dehydration, ketosis, and mineral depletion already discussed. Working out in a sweatsuit is ill advised and merely increases the amount and rate at which all of this occurs.

Starvation and Fasting

Some additional complications that have been reported in individuals who have gone on fasts for more than several days include loss of hair, nutritional deficiencies, gout, potassium depletion, and low blood pressure due to changes in posture and subsequent fainting. Certainly, anybody who is suffering from kidney or heart disease, liver problems, psychiatric problems, and diabetes should avoid fasting like the plague, except under very unusual circumstances and with extremely close supervision in a hospital.

The fasting diets, among which I include the protein sparing fasts, have been responsible for cases of acute intestinal obstruction, in addition to renal failure and lacticacidosis.

Protein-Sparing, Modified Fast

Recently, the author of a widely sold book advocating a pure protein diet asserted that his method was the last opportunity available for those unfortunate individuals who had failed at dieting before—"The Protein-Sparing, Modified Fast." It followed a method used at Harvard, where Dr. George L. Blackburn and his colleagues were doing studies on human nitrogen balance. They were trying to find out the least amount of protein required daily in order to prevent a loss of lean body mass in patients who were fasting.

Let us look at the score card for this rage in dieting. In a strict, university-based study, which generally gets better results because of careful controls, sixty-six percent of the patients kept their weight off for one year, dwindling to thirty-three percent by the end of a year and a half and down to approximately twenty-five percent by the end of two to two and a half years. One of this country's foremost experts on obesity, representing a respected medical institution, commented that it was his feeling that the protein-sparing fast had about the same life expectancy as most of the other programs. One of the dangers, of course, it that people start to treat themselves. One death has been reported: a patient who went on a protein-sparing fast and apparently suffered a heart attack, which was attributed to a lack of potassium caused by this kind of dieting. In fact, one authority stated that he felt that it was the cheating and nibbling by some people on the diet that could be saving their lives. The experts have cautioned patients with kidney disease, previous heart attacks, or liver disease, as well as people with kidney stones and gout, against going on the protein-sparing diet.

I ask you. Are all of these risks worth the less than twenty percent chance of keeping weight off for as long as two years?

Attention Athletes!

A word to athletes of all ages, particularly young athletes. It is commonly thought that eating a high protein diet will increase muscle mass. Muscle mass is increased by exercise and training. You can only utilize the amino acids from protein as quickly as you are able to build muscle tissue through activity. The excess is either converted into glucose for energy or converted into fat for storage. The excess weight that you put on is more fat than muscle. Increased muscle mass and fat may actually hinder rather than improve your physical prowess. Some athletes follow a program in which they load up on carbohydrates during light exercise and eat a low carbohydrate diet during heavy exercise. They believe that by increasing the glycogen content in muscle they will increase their endurance. This may be true, but they are also encouraging the retention of water in muscle in much greater amounts and this may lead to stiffness and discomfort. The excess glycogen may also destroy muscle fiber, and significant changes have also been observed on cardiograms of these individuals.

The "Anti-Cellulite" Diet

A diet that became popular for a while was the "Anti-Cellulite" diet. The diet itself was basically healthy and consisted of lean meats, fish, and poultry, fresh raw vegetables, juice, and six to eight glasses of water a day. It was claimed that this diet would get rid of lumps of fat distributed unevenly over the body, particularly on the thighs. The lumps of fat were referred to as "cellulite." There is only one problem. In thousands of years of medical experience, anatomical dissection, biochemical and physiological investigation, surgical biopsy, and pathological investigation under the microscope, nobody has ever seen or heard of "cellulite."

Vegetarian Diets

In order to be a healthy vegetarian, an individual must be well educated, and as you already know I am in favor of both good health and education. Vegetarian diets, if followed properly, are low in cholesterol and high in fiber and provide the added advantage of costing less. If the vegetarian excludes all foods of animal origin, such as milk, eggs, and cheese, however, then there is a high risk of deficiencies in protein, calcium, iron, Vitamins D and B-12, and folic acid. The strict vegetarian needs expert knowledge and must take in an extensive variety of food.

If you prefer and enjoy a vegetarian diet, be my guest—or rather, be someone else's guest. Vegetarianism can be a problem in your social life, because vegetarian friends are hard to find and your meat-eating friends will often be in an awkward position. The only objections to this kind of diet is that exaggerated claims are made for it and that defi-

ciencies dangerous to your health can occur if it is not practiced knowl-
edgeably.

Vinegar and Seaweed

A diet consisting of vinegar, kelp, lecithin, and Vitamin B-6 was
claimed to be highly successful as long as people stuck to a low calorie
diet. The theory behind the ingestion of kelp (seaweed with lots of iodine)
is that it will stimulate the thyroid and increase metabolism. Exactly the
opposite is true, however. The risk of goiter and thyroid problems may
be increased. Cider vinegar was recommended as a supply of potassium,
which is rarely deficient in our diets and is plentiful in other *more pleasant
foods*. Lecithin has no value in weight control. It is the most abundant
of the phospholipids in foods. Its addition to the diet is superfluous. For
those of you who are irrationally against all additives to food, let me
point out that it is used as an emulsifier in margarine, cheese products,
and processed foods. Lecithin is important in our diets and does play a
role in preventing fatty liver, but it is rarely a deficiency in anyone's diet
and profits the manufacturer, not you. Vitamin B-6 (pyridoxine) must
be the mysterious portion of this diet, as it is a mystery to me why it is
included. It is readily available in our diets, deficiencies are rare, and its
role in dieting is a mystery to research scientists throughout the world.
The Lecithin–B-6–Apple Cider Vinegar–Kelp Diet has been proven to
do nothing about accelerating weight loss, and the quality of this diet
can best be summed up in one word—yecch!

The Zen Diet

The Zen-macrobiotic diets consist of a series of diets numbered
from one to ten. The lower-numbered diets are questionably safe. The
higher you ascend on the scale of diets, the more dangerous they become
as deficiencies in protein, vitamins, and minerals become common. The
macrobiotic diet can result, and has resulted, in death. From a religious
zealot's distorted point of view, death may be desirable in that you get
to meet your maker earlier than intended, but thank goodness most
deeply religious individuals do not think this way. Suicide is a sin, no
matter how you accomplish it.

There is one thing common to most fad diets. They do encourage
you to give up eating. When I was a young boy I used to travel downtown
on the Third Avenue el in New York City for piano lessons. My mother
used to give me thirty-five cents to have dinner, along with the money
for the train fare. I used to cheat a little bit on my dinner by having a
candy bar on my way down to the piano lesson and on the way back.

Then I spent the remainder at the Horn and Hardart Automat, having the most delicious spaghetti, mashed potatoes, and creamed spinach you could imagine. It's a strange thing, but after a year and a half I gave up the piano lessons and the candy bars. I ended up becoming a professional clarinetist and later gave that up for medicine. In all fairness to the people who make candy bars, I lost my taste for them by overindulgence. And so it is with the fad diets. If you were to try the ice cream diet, I am sure that if, after a number of days someone even mentioned the word ice cream, you could be jailed if *contemplated* murder was a crime.

In all honesty, I must admit that all crash diets are a crashing success. The basic reason, which I have already alluded to, is that any diet, if followed, achieves its success primarily through boredom, and I think crash diets should be more appropriately referred to as "boredom diets." One other factor seems to be extremely important and that is the supervision that usually goes along with the diet program. Whether it be the supervision of the book that you are reading, or the physician that you are seeing, or the ever-present, anxious eyes of parents or mates, supervision is crucial. It is with these factors in mind that I came to the conclusion that what we *don't* need is another diet.

PILLS

Following World War II, a breed of doctors sprang up that I refer to as the "Pill Pushers." Some of them are still around, although their pills have changed a bit because of government pressure and withdrawal from the market. Their modus operandi was pretty standard, but had minor variations. For the most part, patients were told that they could eat anything they wanted to eat. They were given a plastic or a cardboard box containing as few as three or as many as twelve different kinds of pills. A typical sample would be as follows:

Thyroid (or one of its derivatives) was provided in doses ranging from one to twelve grains. To give you an idea of what this means, a patient having the thyroid surgically removed for medical reasons would receive an average dose of approximately three grains as total replacement. In other words, some of these diet patients were being given four or more times the amount of thyroid that the body would normally utilize. The results of this practice were a marked increase in the metabolic rate, a heart rate that would go out of sight, symptoms of extreme nervousness, agitation, palpitations, fainting spells, etc. In fact, many patients would suffer thyroid toxicity.

The patient would be provided with *amphetamines* or their derivatives to suppress appetite and also to increase metabolic rate. Some of the symptoms the patient would suffer would be insomnia, extreme nervousness, tremors, and so on.

Diuretics were given to the patient to cause fluid loss. Any excess or superfluous fluid would be lost immediately. Beyond that point, dehydration would begin. The patient would lose vital minerals, particularly potassium, which could result in death.

Laxatives of one sort or another were provided to keep the bowels moving and also to cause an impressive transient loss in weight due to initial emptying of the bowels. Patients would develop a dependency on these laxatives. There was also a risk of irritation of the bowel, loss of vitamins and minerals, and lack of absorption of important food substances because of the rapid transit of food materials through the bowel.

Digitalis was administered primarily to counteract a rapid heart rate caused by the amphetamines and the thyroid. However, giving digitalis to a normal individual poses serious dangers, including toxicity and death. The patient was also given *phenobarbital* or some other barbiturate to counteract the feelings of nervousness caused by the excessive thyroid and amphetamines. The dependency-forming nature of the barbiturates and their possible effects on thinking processes and liver metabolism were all ignored.

Pushing these pills as the basis for dieting, additional medications were employed or substituted. This practice is still going on today. Although the names of some of the medications have been changed and some are no longer used, the dangers are there, if not quite as severe. Patients continue to lose weight, continue to get sick, and ninety-eight percent gain back the weight within two years. The only thing the patients don't get back is the money they shelled out—or their lost health!

Some physicians use one or two medications as a crutch for the demanding patient. Your understanding of what you are asking for may help you keep your mouth shut.

Amphetamines

Using amphetamines will depress the appetite, but within a matter of a few short weeks this effect disappears. Double doses then become necessary in order to maintain the appetite depressant effect. If the individual continues to use the amphetamines, further increase in dosage is required. This creates very serious problems because of the effect of the amphetamines on the nervous system as the tolerance for the drug increases. The problem of drug abuse is less likely to occur with the obese patient because the reason for taking the drug is primarily that of losing weight, but the risk of drug abuse is there nonetheless. This, of course, is in contrast with the "speed freaks" whose motivation is entirely unhealthy, usually a desire to distort the real world and experience a false enhancement of self-image.

Amphetamines and their derivatives have long been used for appetite depression. Because of the problems of habituation, tolerance, and side effects, numerous preparations have appeared on the market. The following is a partial list:

Amphetamine sulfate (Benzedrine)
Benzphetamine Hydrochloride (Didrex)
Dextroamphetamine sulfate (Dexedrine)
Fenfluramine (Pondimin)
Levoamphetamine sulfate and phosphate
Levoamphetamine alginate (Levonor)
Mazindol (Mazanor, Sanorex)
Methamphetamine hydrochloride (Desoxyn, Obetrol)
Phenylpropanolamine (Propadrine, Dexatrim)
Phendemetrazine (Preludin, Plegine, Bontril)
Phentermine (Ionamin, Fastin)
Diethylpropion (Tenuate and Tepanil)

The drug *fenfluramine* is an appetite suppressant which is currently in favor with thousands of physicians and patients. There is no question that this drug does help a patient lose weight by suppressing appetite and the formation of triglycerides, and by stimulating the breakdown of fat and the glucose uptake in muscle. Close to ninety percent of the patients who have taken this drug, however, have reported side effects, and the risk of tolerance also exists.

Most over-the-counter preparations that can be obtained without a prescription contain *phenylpropanolamine*. The effectiveness of this preparation is very questionable, however. Serious reactions to these drugs in otherwise normal patients are relatively rare. Uncomfortable and annoying reactions are very common, nervousness, insomnia, and rapid heart rate being just a few.

Thyroid

The use of hormones in treating obesity is not recommended unless there is a specific proven deficiency in a particular hormone. Otherwise, the effect is to suppress the gland that produces the hormone that is being administered, thus causing atrophy (wasting) and malfunction of that gland. The effects could be disastrous.

Thyroid has enjoyed wide use among physicians for purposes of weight reduction, in spite of the fact that most patients do not have a low thyroid (hypothyroid) condition. When a patient is administered thyroid to aid weight loss, there is usually a temporary increase in the metabolic rate. Because the level of circulating thyroid in the blood returns gradually to the normal state, the physician is then tempted to increase the dosage of thyroid, and usually does, increasing the metabolic rate again, and the cycle occurs over and over again until the patient is taking large doses of thyroid. The patient's own thyroid gland gradually ceases to function. If this is continued for a long period of time, the thyroid will fail to recover. When patients are taken off thyroid after prolonged treatment, they inevitably develop symptoms of hypothyroidism, and it may take weeks or months before they return to a normal state. Unfortunately, many patients who are taking thyroid today will have to take it for the rest of their lives because of this phenomenon. However, new understanding of thyroid metabolism has prompted a reevaluation in the use of thyroid that will be discussed in the chapter on pleasure aids.

Thyroid primarily achieves weight loss by acting on muscle rather than fat. It has been thought that obese individuals who take thyroid are developing a condition that closely resembles a hyperthyroid myopathy (muscle disease) rather than achieving the result that they truly seek.

Metabolic Stimulants

Metabolic stimulants have been used successfully on a temporary basis, but only at great risk. The side reactions are highly toxic and negate their achievements.

Bulk Preparations

Bulk preparations contain methyl-cellulose and have not proven to be effective in weight control to any substantial degree.

HCG

The use of human chorionic gonadotropin (HCG) has received considerable notoriety in the United States and Europe during the past fifteen years. I personally have had extensive experience with the use of this medication until 1973, when the first of several controlled studies of this substance was performed. Several carefully run studies have been done since, and the evidence indicates that HCG contributes nothing to the loss of weight. It is obviously the 500 calorie diet and the close attention given by a physician that accounts for the excellent results, although I still ponder the euphoria and sense of well-being reported by most of my patients (this could be due to the so-called bed-side manner effect). No studies evaluating the psychological or emotional effects of the usage of HCG have been done, to my knowledge.

BEHAVIORAL TREATMENT OF OBESITY

At the Medical University of South Carolina a team of behavioral scientists conducted a ten week course in behavioral modification for 165 female, chronically obese patients. Many of these patients had other medical complications. The following results were obtained:

144 completed the ten week course. Of these, only sixty-four followed through for twelve months. Eight of these patients were lost to follow-up evaluation. Of the remaining fifty-six, six had kept their weight off, eleven continued to lose weight, and thirty-nine had regained their weight and more. One medical journal commented editorially, "If a talented, devoted, and able team of psychologists and allied behavioral scientists achieved no better than the above results, the cost-benefit of such efforts is questionable and physicians should be realistic in their recommendations."

The current state of the art leaves much to be desired. Is there a future in it? I doubt it. Maybe 1984 and brainwashing will change that.

SURGERY

The jejuno-ileal by-pass procedure has been reserved for individuals who are at least 100 pounds overweight, preferably under fifty years of age, who have been unsuccessful in losing weight, and to whom weight loss is critically necessary for medical and psychiatric purposes. An operative mortality of about five percent has been reported. Complications such as malnutrition, mineral and vitamin deficiency, as well as some neurological difficulties have been reported. Long-term survival of these patients may be in jeopardy, but the answer will not be forthcoming for several decades.

JAWS

An illustration of the extremes to which people will go in order to lose weight is the method of having the jaws wired shut by the local dentist so that eating is impossible. The individual can only sip fluids through a straw. Most patients going on this very drastic approach do lose weight, although I knew one patient who gained weight because she was grinding up all sorts of things in the blender and drinking four to five malts a day. Even if the liquids to be ingested comprise a well-balanced portion of carbohydrates, proteins, fats, minerals, and vitamins, I advise my patients strongly against making the attempt and warn them of the possible dangers. In addition, this method has the same problem I have referred to over and over again; the individual *learns* nothing and will gain the weight back, and the net result will be the same.

DIETS FROM THE NUTRITION EXPERTS

It is absolutely amazing that most of the popular "nutrition experts" lack a formal education in their field, have no degrees to back up their training, and fail to cite sources for the materials and statistics that they use in their writings. Very often, if they do extract material from legitimate research journals, medical journals, or standard texts, it is taken out of context, distorted, exaggerated to extremes, and then twisted to suit their own imaginations.

Unhealthy food for the brain often leads to unhealthy food for the belly. When reading books by so-called authorities on nutrition, it is always wise to check their credentials, background, and training. Unfortunately, this may not always be a safeguard against misinformation, distortion, and dangerous advice.

ORGANIC FOODS

Whether food is organically grown or not is not the most important question. What you eat and how much you eat is. Investigations by government laboratories have revealed, for example, that the levels of pesticides in our regular food are not too different from levels in "organic food." Comparisons between artificial fertilizer and natural fertilizers might shock some people. For example, natural phosphate rock used in organic farming may contain toxic levels of fluorine. Interestingly enough, if this rock is processed to be used as a chemical fertilizer, the fluorine is removed. In this instance, therefore, the artificial fertilizer would be better than the natural fertilizer. Despite detailed comparisons between chemical fertilizers and natural fertilizers such as compost or animal manure, however, the substances which plants ultimately use in order to grow are chemicals such as potassium, magnesium, ammonia, nitrates, etc. These are basically inorganic chemical substances, regardless of their source. The plants, by utilizing these chemicals, as well as water, carbon dioxide, and sunlight, create the carbohydrates, fats, proteins and minerals that we have discussed. Most foods grown today are somewhat

mineral deficient and most people would benefit by taking a multivitamin–mineral supplement.

Vitamin C is ascorbic acid, and ascorbic acid, regardless of where
it comes from, is ascorbic acid. The chemical atomic formula is the same.
The food alarmists have made millions on their warnings about con-
cocted, imaginary hazards and have neuroticized countless thousands or
even millions with their fear tactics. The health food industry and its
proponents continually make unsubstantiated, unprovable claims of health
benefits for their products. They constantly debase and degrade ordinary
foods with exaggeration, distortion, and outright lies. Similarly, to point
to a single additive, pesticide, or chemical that has been shown to be
dangerous and then to extend that statement to include all chemicals,
additives, or pesticides, is irresponsible. The benefits derived from these
substances in providing us with plentiful, nutritious, tasty, and inexpen-
sive foods far outweigh any of the proven damage that may have been
caused by a few exceptions. Let no one distort my meaning by intimating
that I don't care whether a substance is safe or not. I do strongly advocate
constant vigilance and honest, meaningful, scientific research in the production and processing of anything that comes in contact with our lives.

SUGAR

What about that old devil, sugar?

As you recall, table sugar is sucrose, and sucrose is composed of
one unit each of glucose and fructose. We know that glucose is the basic
product in the metabolism and utilization of carbohydrates by the body.
The phony experts and nutritionists would have you believe that honey
and molasses are far superior to sugar. Well, honey is a mixture of
glucose and fructose just as table sugar is, and molasses is a by-product
of sugar refining. The major difference lies in the vitamin and mineral
content. If an individual eats a fairly well-balanced diet, then the vitamins
and minerals contained in honey and molasses should be provided in
more adequate amounts by other foods. The major problem with any
of these substances is excessive intake at the expense of other foods. The
calories from carbohydrates are the same regardless of the source. The
problem of obesity and tooth decay can develop just as readily from
honey as it can from sugar. So the key word again is *moderation*. Oh yes,
please brush your teeth after each meal. The claims for predigested
enzyme and hormone content of honey are totally irrelevant because
these products are broken down, digested, converted, and utilized as
glucose and are certainly not absorbed in their original state.

So, if you've stopped eating sugar like the faddists tell you to and are using honey instead, I think you're wasting your time, unless you like honey better!

COFFEE

In studying some of the claims of the food faddists, let's look at the problem of coffee. A fatal dose of caffeine, which is a major ingredient in coffee, is estimated to be approximately ten grams. This would be equivalent to between 70 and 100 cups of coffee. Experiments done with large numbers of people indicate that, as with so many other substances, the tolerance of each individual differs. The symptoms of insomnia and restlessness should serve as indications of an individual's tolerance. Caffeine is cautioned against, for example, for people with peptic ulcers, because it stimulates gastric secretion. Ulcers are obviously not *caused* by the food we eat, however, because if they were, everybody in Italy would have an ulcer. We have more ulcers in the United States than they do in Italy. Interestingly enough, some studies have shown that coffee has been beneficial for people with a condition called gastroesophageal reflux. This condition causes the acid to reflux from the stomach up into the swallowing tube, the esophagus. There is even great controversy as to whether or not it is the caffeine in the coffee that causes some of the problems which have been attributed to it. More than one hundred different components have been identified in coffee. Caffeine, however, has some beneficial effects. It does appear to stimulate rapid and clear flow of thought and does seem to relieve the symptoms of fatigue or drowsiness. Motor activity of the body is enhanced, enabling an individual to work faster with fewer errors in certain tasks. There seems to be a statistical relationship between the ingestion of caffeine and the incidence of bladder cancer in women, however, although no causal relationship has been established. It didn't seem to make a difference whether the coffee was weak or strong, instant or regular, decaffeinated or not, or whether the individual used sugar or nonsugar sweeteners. The facts as they now stand, based on careful controlled studies, do not show a cause and effect relationship.

Irresponsible statements by self-appointed "experts" based on nothing more than old wives' tales and imagination are not to be compared with intensive hard work based on sound scientific principles. The important word for the problem of excessive ingestion is the same as it would be for any other food, *moderation*. Do you really have to drink coffee?

There is some evidence that coffee is associated with an increased risk of death from coronary disease, an increased incidence of cardiac arrythmias, birth defects, fibrocystic disease of the breast, bladder cancer, and pancreatic cancer.

WHOLE GRAINS AND CEREALS

If you enjoy whole grains and unrefined cereals, by all means eat them and enjoy them. They do contain vitamins and minerals, carbohydrates, proteins, fats, and fiber. If, however, you don't enjoy them, don't be frightened, don't feel you're going to be cheated out of long life. Almost all processed grains are enriched by the addition of some vitamins and minerals, but these do not replace all that are taken out. To most people, they taste much better. Now, I happen to love an english muffin once in a while, or maybe some french toast made with thick, fluffy white bread, and I enjoy a piece of soft, moist, delicious chocolate cake and quite a few other delectable items that are made from refined flour (*in moderation,* of course). I firmly believe in a healthy diet, but I also believe in a delicious diet. I believe that life was meant to be enjoyed; that fate confronts us with enough calamities and disappointments; that finding pleasure, safely, wherever we can, is a legitimate pursuit of happiness. The food faddists are not completely wrong. They say that these foods are bad for you. I say that too much is bad for you. Why not substitute whole grains as much as is possible and practical for you?

VITAMINS AND MEGAVITAMINS

Generally, megadoses of vitamins are unnecessary and will not help you to lose weight. Let's take a look at the so-called megadose vitamin supplements and the "Live-forever-cure-everything-with-huge-doses-of-vitamins" sect. Two vitamins, E and C in particular, have received more notoriety and attention than any other two substances in history. In fact, for a while I thought they were going to take the place of sex and night baseball.

Vitamin E

Since 1946 when Vitamin E was first touted as a miracle vitamin, all kinds of sensational claims have been made for it. Most notably, it was supposed to be of great benefit in cases of allergy, asthma, arthritis, skin diseases of all kinds, vascular problems, heart disease and sexual problems, to name a few. Vitamin E is so plentiful in our foods (see the chapter on foods) that we would have no need for doctors if all of these claims were true. Serious investigation by research and medical institutions all over the world have been carried out. The net result is that none of the claims for Vitamin E have been substantiated, and in fact, comparative studies with patients who received *placebos* (inert capsules containing harmless powder) reported marvelous results equaling the claims of the "E" faddists.

When Vitamin E was intentionally withheld from the diet of experimental animals, muscular problems developed in guinea pigs, chicks, and rabbits; retardation in growth and reproduction, as well as liver problems, occurred in rats; and heart damage occurred in calves. But these difficulties have never turned up in man under experimental conditions, and the probable invalidity of direct parallels shows up in the fact that the chicks didn't develop what rats developed, calves didn't develop what guinea pigs developed, and so on.

If you're going to believe that the effects on experimental animals directly parallel those in human beings, then at least be aware of the fact that excessive intake of Vitamin E can be *toxic* (deadly) to animals. All of the conditions that have been observed in animals in which Vitamin E deficiency has been produced have been tested for in people without positive results. The following represent the facts as they are known today:

Notice to patients taking anticoagulants: You should be extremely cautious about taking any extra Vitamin E at all. Although there is some evidence that Vitamin E may be beneficial in cases of peripheral vascular disease, excessive Vitamin E can produce hypertension.

Vitamin E appears to protect the lipid in red blood cell membranes from peroxidation (the formation of toxic free radicals), which produces degeneration of tissue. Selenium and Vitamin E work synergistically and act as anti-oxidants.

Vitamin A

Enlargement of the skull (water on the brain) has been attributed to an overdose of Vitamin A given to infants. Even relatively small doses of Vitamin A (25,000–50,000 IU) when given over a period of a month or more, have been known to cause symptoms of nausea, vomiting, weakness, ringing in the ears, double vision, headaches, eye damage, and even blindness. Other symptoms attributed to prolonged use of Vitamin A include anemia, liver enlargement, jaundice, spleen enlargement, abdominal pain, joint and muscle pain, brittle nails, dry skin, and loss of hair.

Vitamin C

Some evidence exists to indicate that individuals who stay on large doses of Vitamin C develop an efficient mechanism in their bodies to destroy the excess. Unfortunately, when they stop taking the large doses of Vitamin C, that mechanism will persist and patients may have to take large doses of Vitamin C for the rest of their lives because of an ever-present deficiency. The excessive intake of ascorbic acid (Vitamin C) may be responsible for an increase in the incidence of urinary tract stones among patients with gout and also in the development of oxalate stones among normal patients. Large doses of Vitamin C may also cause the destruction of B-12. On the positive side, however, Vitamin C appears to reduce the duration and severity of the common cold.

Niacin

Large doses of niacin inhibit cardiac muscle metabolism, cause injury to the liver cells, interfere with the flow of bile, and cause skin discoloration, elevation of blood sugar and blood uric acid levels, peptic ulcers, and gouty arthritis. On the positive side, niacin (Nicotinic Acid) is believed to be a preventive in peripheral vascular disease. It lowers plasma cholesterol and triglycerides. Tryptophan is also converted into nicotinic acid; therefore, if tryptophan intake is low, more niacin is needed.

Niacin plays a strong role as a coenzyme component in cellular respiration. The lack of niacin gives rise to many neurological and psychological problems.

GOODBYE MR. FAD

The single most important objection to any crash diet is that it changes nothing, not even your weight, because the weight loss is too temporary to count. Medical evidence indicates that obese individuals who continually lose and regain weight develop a progressive increase in blood cholesterol and lipid levels. The demoralization and disillusionment that comes from this process is even more damaging.

What have any of these diets and nutritional myths taught us? Even though we have lost weight with them, have we learned anything? Can we stick to any of these diets for the rest of our lives comfortably or safely? I don't have to answer that question because the public already has. Only two percent of all dieters achieve long-term success with any of these diets.

Where do we go from here?

On the one hand we have the hucksters peddling their miracle diets, duping and ripping-off the public with potentially dangerous, unrewarding, unsuccessful treatments. Strangely enough, on the other hand we have the dedicated, sincere scientist whose dispassionate presentation of therapeutic requirements yields no better result.

A recent consensus indicates that there are three basic requirements for a good diet: One, that it provide proper nutrition; two, that it satisfy a person's cultural needs; and three, that it fulfill a person's pyschological needs.

The Pleasure Principle does this.

Scene 2
Fuel for Thought—
How We Got This Way

*What we need even more than foresight or
hindsight, is insight. Foresight tells us what is
coming, hindsight tells us what has happened, but
insight gives us the opportunity to change.*

As I recall, it was at a New Years' Eve party that Joe the Glut agreed
to be hypnotized. Every year, Lodge 32 of the Fraternal Order of the
Bellowing Geese welcomed in the new year at the local country club.
The entertainment that year was provided by a stage hypnotist named
Morton the Magnificent. Little did anyone realize that the events that
were about to take place would be recounted on national television and
make the headlines of newspapers throughout the country. The town
of Klutsville would soon be mentioned in a hundred languages all over
the globe.

When Morton the Magnificent asked for a volunteer from the audience, Joe the Glut was persuaded by his friends (with very little urging,
I might add) to offer himself as a subject. Morton the Magnificent es-
corted Joe to the middle of the stage, where he seated Joe in a comfortable armchair. He placed his index finger on Joe's forehead and told
Joe to look up at his finger. He then suggested to Joe that his eyes were
getting very heavy and that they would close, which they did. He then
told Joe that his body was getting very heavy, his breathing would intensify, and he would go into a deep hypnotic trance. It was obvious to
everyone in the audience that the hypnosis was working, because Joe
immediately began snoring very loudly. Morton the Magnificent had to

suggest to Joe that his trance would be a silent one. Joe gave a couple of snorts and his breathing became quiet. Morton the Magnificent then announced to the audience that he would take Joe back in time to another life, to an age long since forgotten. He then described to Joe how he was being transported through the ethereal vapors of time back to a different world, one hidden in the far reaches of his mind. "Another time, another place . . . another time, another place . . . another time, another place . . . ." He then asked Joe, "Where are you now?" Joe's voice came over the microphone in a slightly higher pitch and with a thick foreign accent, Slavic in character, "I am by the strumine." An audible murmur rippled through the audience. Someone in the audience called out, "That's Polish for 'river.'" Morton then asked, "Who are you?" Again, the strange voice answered, "Count Andrew Rajevel." Morton the Magnificent's voice cracked with excitement. "What are you doing at the strumine?" he asked. "I am waiting for Anastasia," answered Joe. The murmur of the audience now became a "strumine" itself. "Who is Anastasia?" asked Morton. "She is my swadny smotyl, my skoham," Joe answered. Again, someone in the audience said, "That's Polish for 'pretty butterfly' and 'love.'" The audience was now in a frenzy. Several women fainted, half the men in the audience were pouring themselves stiff drinks. The strange voice came over the microphone again, "Burnotka jevchinka shwa jevo vlas . . . anyo ya tom viedja book som vibrow chas . . ." Morton turned to the audience and asked, "Does anyone know what that means?" Someone in the audience called out, "It's about a little girl 'Burnotka' walking through the woods, and something about angels taking her to meet God." At this point, the audience started to get so out of hand, that Morton raised his arms high in the air and shouted, "You are now being transported back to the present. When I count to three, you will wake up and you will be here *now*, in Klutsville." With that, Morton counted to three and Joe opened his eyes. Seeing all of the commotion and thinking the time was right, Joe shouted, "Happy New Year!" and ran off the stage to embrace his wife.

During the next few hectic days there were television interviews, continuous questions from newspaper reporters, the telephone ringing incessantly, and thousands of sightseers from all over the country driving past Joe's house. Joe's mother sat, strangely quiet, on the back porch through all of this as if she herself were in a trance. Joe was convinced of his immortality, of reincarnation, and believed that he possessed secret powers (if he could only find them). Joe made himself a small fortune on the exclusive interviews, television appearances, and on the royalties to a book that somebody else wrote called *Joe's Jubilant Journey*.

When all of the excitement finally subsided, Joe suddenly became aware of his mother's silence. For over six weeks his mother had been sitting in a rocking chair on the back porch, from sunup to sundown, staring off into the distance without uttering a word. When the last interviews had ended and the tourists disappeared, Joe's mother quietly got up from the rocking chair and started to go about her long overdue housework. She soon began to hum a tune while she worked and everyone in the family relaxed, assured that Joe's mother would recover from the shock of all that had happened. There was something strange about her humming because it almost sounded as if she were an amused child. A melodious chuckle from sunrise to sunset filled the house. Oh, if they could only know what was going on in that little old lady's thoughts. If they could only know that Mrs. Glut was thinking of the time, forty years earlier, when little Joe was three years old. She remembered very clearly that the Polish maid they had hired to take care of Joe used to carry him around on her shoulders and tell him charming little stories. Joe's favorite was about a Count who lived by a river and waited for his pretty, beloved "butterfly" named Anastasia. In her thickly accented, slightly high-pitched voice, the maid would sing the same little Polish poem that Joe had sung on stage the night he was hypnotized.

MIND, MATTER, OR MAGIC?

There is no magic in this world, and there are very few accidents. If you are overweight, it is no accident. Human behavior evolves and it begins when life begins. Every moment of life is an experience and every experience is a teacher. At this very moment you represent the sum total of your life's happenings. The manner in which each experience affects your life is determined by your awareness and by all that has happened to you up until the moment. Your brain has recorded everything, and like Joe the Glut, you recall childhood incidents in later life. They may expose or impose themselves many years later in the same distorted form in which they were perceived by the child's mind. How did we get fat? We overate! Why did we overeat? Now that is the real question. Let's see if we can seek out the "Polish maid" of our obesity.

There are basically two kinds of obese patients for whom reducing therapy has failed. One group of patients lose weight and then quickly gain it back over and over again. They have been referred to by some doctors as "yo-yo syndrome" patients. This is by far the largest and most common group. Another group of patients lose very little weight or none at all, continuing to stay fat or simply getting fatter. There are basically two groups of obese patients who are successful. These groups are rarely more than thirty pounds overweight, are successful in losing weight and keeping it off, or may fluctuate weight gradually. We have already discussed some of the physiological and regulatory disturbances that may be playing a role in the difficulties encountered in trying to keep the weight off. The patients with serious weight problems who have failed to either take the weight off in substantial amounts, or who keep fluctuating up and down by large degrees, eventually end up seeking psychiatric help when all other medical approaches have failed. Hilde Bruch, M.D., a Professor of Psychiatry at Baylor College of Medicine in Houston, Texas, has written an excellent book entitled *Eating Disorders: Obesity, Anorexia Nervosa and the Person Within* (Basic Books Incorporated). Dr. Bruch points out that some patients function better when they are obese. For these patients, obesity becomes a mechanism by which they protect themselves against more serious illness. In essence, it represents an ineffective attempt to stay healthy. As an individual develops, however, obesity may become an inappropriate but habitual response to problems, and the pattern becomes deeply embedded as the pressures and insults of life grow. Because the patients do not realize the mechanisms involved, they cannot comfortably shed the protective layer of fat. Their hunger is excessive, they develop anxieties and have great difficulty in functioning in everyday life. Dr. Bruch points out that the individuals who are most affected and hurt by the insults of a society that condemn overweight are those who suffer from "severe self-doubt and have a poor body image and an inadequate self-concept and consequently develop extreme dependence on the opinion of others in all areas of living, not only in regard to weight and appearance." She points out that when these individuals try to reduce, "they feel diminished and empty and become even more unhappy." Cultural condemnation is only part of the problem. The family's attitude and environment during a child's early years appears to play a more significant role. Rejection early in life, for example, leaves a deep scar that may fester and create serious psychological problems in later life.

There is no single psychological classification for the obese. Each case must be carefully considered by itself and thorough investigation into a person's background is necessary. The purpose of this chapter is to familiarize you with the mechanisms and circumstances that most frequently cause obesity. When obesity begins early in life and then continues, individuals frequently feel that they are not in control of their own bodies. It is interesting that the feelings of these individuals correlate strongly with the self-perceptions of poor and underprivileged social classes who feel that they lack control of their lives, groups in which the incidence of obesity is also higher.* Obesity becomes the excuse for their problems rather than the result of their problems. They do not understand that they are fat because they have felt unloved. They feel that they are unloved because they are fat. This situation generates other negative feelings, and they fail to socialize or communicate well with the world around them. The chances of permanent weight loss are slim (no pun intended) without understanding, dealing with, and changing their inner feelings. Should a person be successful in losing weight and remaining slender, the other emotional difficulties and behavior patterns may become more intense. For this reason the Pleasure Principle goes beyond the concept of just losing, and keeping weight off. The concept of *pleasure with self* becomes a primary target, an absolute necessity. Losing weight may make you appear beautiful, but you still might *feel* unattractive. You may look thin, but *feel* fat; look exciting, but still *feel* dull. You look happy, but *feel* miserable; appear outgoing, but *feel* alone; appear confident, but *feel* uncertain. While you appear carefree and content, you *feel* troubled, sad, dissatisfied, unlucky, and abandoned. The feelings that you have about your life are the essence of a healthy existence; appearance should be its reflection, not its substitute or cover-up.

Ever since Freud contributed his monumental thinking and concepts to the understanding of the role of emotions and its relation to disease, there has been a tendency to separate the mind and body in both theory and practice. The mind is simply a concept representing the nonphysical funtioning of the brain. The mind may be talked about as though it were a separate entity, but it is an integral part of the brain just as the fluid characteristics of water are an integral part of the water itself. Patients are constantly asking their doctors, "Is this mental or physical?" Doctors who answer that question fall into the trap of fostering the unfair separation of the two. As research progresses, we are establishing that there are not two entities, but only one. Thoughts and emotions are products of a complex biochemical, electrical, and physiological phenomenon which responds to all forms of outside stimuli. Different chemical substances have been discovered in the brain in larger amounts in the presence of certain emotions, and certain chemicals have been synthesized which, when ingested, enhance or block chemical reactions

---

*An interesting correlation has been pointed out between minority groups and obese children. Both groups seem to be obsessed with their life situations, and exhibit the characteristics of passivity, a sense of rejection, and withdrawal. This results in isolation from society and an unhappy existence, in addition to progressive inactivity.

in the brain, thus changing the emotional feelings and/or ability to think.

Obesity is a medical condition, but it can be correlated with cultural and personal factors. Society, however, strongly resists the idea that individual emotions and even the attitudes of the society itself, are major factors in the cause of disease. It is no wonder then that patients want to believe that their obesity is due to a sluggish metabolism, a low thyroid, some glandular disturbance, or maybe even the "tooth fairy". Obesity, we have learned, is more common the lower you go on the economic scale. Why do the wealthy tend to be slim and the poor tend to be fat? Does it have to do with economic stress and the relative ability to control one's fate? What about food as a symbol? I seem to recall in my professional and social experience that poor individuals usually offer more food to their visitors and guests than do the wealthy. Is overeating a means by which the poor can mask their deprivation, or hide scarcity with an obvious show of abundance? Understanding one's self, and what we have become, may help us in achieving our goals and in maintaining them.

Why is obesity so difficult to treat? Why do we gain weight? Why do we make ourselves look so unattractive? Why are common, everyday activities so difficult to do? Why do we encourage others to look at us with disapproval, condemn us with their words, and ridicule us in their thoughts? Why do we gain weight when it robs us of sexual expression, better jobs, and self-respect? Why is it so difficult to lose weight when to do so would improve our health, prevent disease, restore our self-respect, and increase life's opportunities?

It is frequently mentioned in medical literature that obesity is a complex disorder. Obesity encompasses the total life history, and physical being of an individual. We have already covered the biochemical, physiological, and anatomical aspects of this disorder; we also know that the genetic background, the medical history, and the physical functioning of an individual's body all play an important role. However, obesity is one condition in which the psychological development and behavior patterns play an equally significant, or even greater, role. It appears too, from most of the work that has been done in the field of psychology, that there are almost as many variations of etiology (cause) as there are people. If you remember, I showed you in earlier chapters what I believe to be a fairly complete history form that should be used when dealing with the problems of obesity. The purpose of such a form is to highlight the possible origins and reinforcing factors of obesity in a patient's life. It is hoped that when you understand the emotional factors, behavioral patterns, and environmental influences that brought about and perpetuated obesity, you might then gain the motivation, understanding, and direction necessary to become slender. When insight and motivation are combined with a practical, ongoing, nonsacrificial diet, most patients will lose weight and keep it off.

ROOTS AND REASONS

There are two major psychological theories on obesity.

The classical psychodynamic school of thought, originated by Freud, speaks of internal drives, one which seeks to satisfy the need for nurturing. These drives are essential, and are innate, or inborn. For example, hunger* is considered a drive that is necessary to satisfy the need for food that keeps the organism alive and is, therefore, essential for life. If the drive is not fulfilled, the organism dies. The need for love is also a basic drive; if unmet, the need can, according to some experimentation, also result in death. There is, however, a significant difference between these two drives. There can be no substitute for food. Love, on the other hand, can sometimes be satisfied (though inappropriately) by other things. Sadly, the "other thing" is often food. The organism may survive, but emotionally it is undernourished and physically it is overnourished.

The other major school of psychological thinking is referred to as the "associative" or "conditioning" school. The proponents of this concept rely more upon environmental factors to explain psychological phenomena. They believe that eating patterns are set by early experience, and therefore, love and feeding would be closely associated by the organism because both are provided by the mother to the infant. They believe that the patterns for eating will be further influenced or conditioned by the teaching and examples set by the parents for the growing child. Both basic concepts are probably operative and play significant roles in personality and behavior development. The difference appears to be essentially one of focus. With this alliance of concepts in mind, let us proceed.

Investigation of the physical and psychological causes of obesity has revealed only a handful of diseases. Among the relatively small number

---

*In common usage, the words *hunger* and *appetite* are used interchangeably. However, I will use the term *hunger* to indicate the feeling of the need for food, either physiological or psychological, or a combination of both. Hunger is an instinctual drive. It is a physiological signal of the body that tells us there is a need for food. There is great evidence that it even signals the type of food that is needed. *Appetite*, on the other hand, is more a feeling that we get in response to past experiences and emotions. It involves food preferences based on our taste and the pleasures that we get from eating foods.

of cases, control of the obesity is relatively simple and successful, that is, when a cure is available. However, the overwhelming majority of obesity cases are emotionally based. Family and social environments establish (and constantly reinforce) the behavioral pattern of eating.

The term *oral gratification* is used in psychology to describe pleasure obtained through stimulation of the mouth and tastebuds, and the satisfaction of the sensation of appetite. It is accepted as the first focus or center for gratification in the development of the child. The earliest and most primitive reflex in the infant is the sucking movement of the mouth. It can easily be seen in a newborn baby by simply stroking the baby's cheek. The baby's head will turn toward the finger and the sucking movements of the lips and the mouth are activated (the rooting reflex). Stimulation of the mouth with a nipple and the insertion of liquid and food quiet the crying of the child, bringing apparent contentment and restful sleep. A crucial ingredient in this situation is physical contact with the infant. The infant must be held while it is fed or it may not survive in spite of the food. This is heavily reinforced as we travel through life's different stages, in a thousand different ways, over and over again. Is it any wonder that we bite our nails, reach for something to eat, grab a cigarette or suck on a pencil when we are upset and under pressure?

It becomes clear that food, which satisfies that well-ingrained need for oral gratification, can become a substitute for a wide variety of emotions. Suppose you were angry and were unable to express that anger, because there was no one around to express it to. What if expressing your anger would cause you greater problems? Maybe you were afraid to express the anger? Food could become the pacifier, the means by which you would calm your anxiety. The feelings of anger would be suppressed. Eating becomes an adaptive mechanism, a way of handling emotional stress.

Sublimation is the term used to describe a healthy defensive technique developed by the individual against these overwhelming feelings and events. Work, hobbies, sports and other healthy diversionary activities are examples of sublimation—a healthy means of coping. However, insight, understanding, and intellectual awareness are the most powerful weapons available to us. The unhealthy techniques or defenses used by obese individuals are what we commonly refer to as excuses. Workers in the field of psychotherapy categorize these defenses under such terms as denial, projection, displacement, rationalization and reaction-formation. In certain instances these techniques can be extremely helpful if used properly. Eating as a defense is ultimately unhealthy. For our purposes, the following quotes will give you a pretty good idea of the unhealthy ways we deal with obesity and why they result in failure:

"It won't make a difference . . ."	(When it really will make a difference.)
"I'll just have a taste . . ."	(And you end up eating the whole bowl.)
"It's all Henry's fault and I . . ."	(Henry got you upset [you let Henry upset you], but he didn't make you eat the whole pie.)
"I was so upset, I didn't know what I was doing and I . . ."	(You ate a gallon of ice cream, five pizzas, and a pickle—and you didn't know what you were doing?)
"I couldn't do it because . . ."	(It was Aunt Sofie's 85th birthday on Monday, the PTA meeting on Tuesday, the Klutsville Homeowner's Association on Wednesday . . .)

In all fairness, let's "give the devil his due." Psychotherapists understand most of this behavior is unconscious, but, if you could have the insight, understanding, and awareness immediately before you got into trouble, wouldn't it help? This is where the Pleasure Principle comes in. Be patient, we're getting there!

MIXED-UP MESSAGES

The experiences of development are as numerous and different as the population. Obese people have basic, common characteristics in their background, but no two people are alike. Generally speaking, however, in the obese person, the physiological signals of the body have been maladapted, distorted and confused. Healthy programming of hunger, and an awareness of its appropriate pathways, is blocked and the faulty programming leads to the intake of food, when in fact, it is another *nonnutritional* need that cries out to be filled. Anxiety, depression, frustration, anger, guilt, and the need for love, are all common feelings that the individual incorrectly learns to satisfy by eating. *The impulse to eat is brought about by the wrong need.* Satisfaction is usually temporary and the process repeats itself because the true need has not been filled.

When such individuals are placed in a hospital or clinic, under strict control, they are successful in losing weight. The removal of stress may be the key factor. When the controls are removed, the patient regains the weight.

As a child develops during the early months of life, the mother is the most significant factor in the environment. Her reaction to her child's behavior has a profound influence on that child's development. The mother's behavior patterns, are, of course, determined by her own development. It is impossible for her to hide her own emotional state, including her own unhealthy responses to the stresses of life, from (and including) the growing infant. To a significant degree, the infant's environment can strongly interfere with the child's future ability to distinguish between physiological (body) needs, emotional needs, and an appropriate behavioral response for either. For example, if the infant is fed at what appears to be appropriate times, and in response to what appears to be appropriate signals of hunger, then most likely a fitting relationship between body needs and feeding will develop. If, however, the infant is fed in an erratic manner, totally unrelated to body needs and in amounts that are equally unsuited for the occasions, whether they be too large or too small, then the child's future eating habits will likely follow a similar pattern. Confused, inappropriate, excessive, and extreme will best describe the adult whose early learning processes lacked a proper identification with the body's biological needs. Imagine for a moment, the possible future effects of the following situations involving infant feeding:

> Forced feeding at a time when the food is not wanted.
> Neglect or withholding of food when the infant cries out for nourishment.
> Feeding the infant whenever it cried, regardless of the reason.

The learning process through the interaction of the child and its environment becomes more complex as the child grows. The individual may never learn to recognize the symptoms of physiological hunger, that is, the body's way of signaling the basic physiological needs for nourishment.

There are two basic aspects to the phenomenon referred to as hunger: the physical need for food and the emotional need for food. In medical and psychological terms they are often referred to as psychological hunger. A theoretical discussion of order, origin, or importance will not help us understand or combat the problem of obesity. For our purposes, recognizing that the phenomenon of hunger involves many things, and then looking at the more common experiences which occur and have an influence on obesity, will serve to give us some insight into your own situation.

For example, if you learn some of the more common reasons why people have a tendency to become obese, then you will take the next step and try to identify some of the events in your life that have contributed to your problem. If through recognizing the origin of your problem you can see that the behavior is misdirected and destructive, you will be on your guard whenever such behavior starts (and the Pleasure Principle will help you do this). You can then make a conscious, intelligent, controlled, healthy decision to lose or maintain your weight and enjoy your life more fully than ever before.

To reiterate, hunger not only involves the physical or physiological signal of the body, it also represents a composite response of feelings, emotions, and experiences. A major problem arises when the individual is unable to distinguish the hunger drive that comes from the physiological needs of the body, from the emotional associations and conditioning that occur during the years of development.

Let us trace some hypothetical, but common representative examples of situations that follow us through life. They form patterns and then are reinforced over and over again. They become a part of us. An inner-driving force, a ghost out of the past, expressing itself through the unconscious, and dictating silently the way we react to life here and now.

THIS IS YOUR LIFE!

What It's Like to Be Born

Life begins in a warm tub bath. Most of the time there is sleep. At other times there are sounds, constant sounds. There is a rhythmic thumping that goes on and on. Then there are gurgling sounds, sometimes low pitched, sometimes high pitched. You seem to be constantly in motion. Most of it is pleasant and you seem to sway gently back and forth. You are warm and secure. But sometimes there are sudden jarring movements. Occasionally, there is a harsh or loud sound. It seems to make you vibrate and the feeling is unpleasant. There is no need to breathe and no need to eat. Just sounds, movement, and feelings of warmth.

Gradually, you begin to feel pressure. The pressure is around your head and then you feel your entire body being squeezed. The squeezing comes and goes; becomes more intense and more rapid. The pressure around your head becomes almost unbearable. You are being crushed! Then your head is being pulled. Then your body is being crushed and suddenly, an explosion! A cold whiteness envelops you. Your legs are being pulled, the lower part of your back stings with sudden blows. Something is stuck into your nose and your mouth. Your body is being jarred mercilessly. Something strange happens to you all over and you open your mouth and hear sounds coming from within you and you feel as if your insides are trying to reach outside of you. You feel as though you are being pulled from all sides, turned and twisted. The warmth, the quiet, the pleasant sounds, are gone now. There is only the cold, harsh brightness. You feel the coldness coming in through your face, then into your body, and you are aware of your mouth. It is a strange feeling, it is as if you want to take that old warmth, softness, and security into your mouth. Then, after an eternity, something warm and soft surrounds you. It is not quite as good as before, but it's a lot better than the cold and harshness.

After the many hours of labor and delivery, the umbilical cord is severed and the source of nutrition obtained from your mother's circulation is cut off. The gastrointestinal tract begins to take over. The nervous system and the body chemistry intensify their work and the early reflexes of sucking and rooting begin. Touching the infant's cheek causes the head to turn in that direction, the lips reach out, and the sucking motion begins. As the need for nourishment increases, the gastrointestinal system is signalled. There is an increased movement in the intestines, saliva flows in the mouth, and the muscular activity of the lips, the cheek, and the jaws begin.

If not responded to, these activities of the gastrointestinal tract become uncomfortable and painful and the infant responds by crying. The infant is alone, out of its cocoon. There is no gentle, sloshing, warm fluid to massage and caress. Now, there are strange, uncomfortable sensations, occurring from within and without. When the infant cries, warm, gentle touchings to the skin occur and a pleasant tasting fluid is placed in the mouth. It flows into the body and calms the contractions of the intestinal tract. *It imparts a feeling of security and tranquillity. Something placed in the mouth has made the world right.*

Then there are times when something is not placed in the mouth and the pains get worse. The turmoil of the body increases, the reactions of the infant intensify. The face gets red, the arms and legs move wildly. Its cries become more severe. Only when food is placed in the mouth and the child is held and comforted, does the terrible ordeal come to an end.

Early Childhood

Scene: Early Morning. Mother in her nightgown and robe, cleaning up the kitchen. Big brother and sister just went off to school. Daddy left for work and . . . little sister (two years old) comes into the kitchen, she climbs up onto the chair and reaches onto the table for a small glass of orange juice. As two-year-olds often will, she knocks over the glass . . . Mother, harried and tired, turns around and shouts, "Can't you do anything right? You'll be the death of me!"

The words and the scene are long since forgotten, but the feelings remain. "You can't do anything right. You'll be the death of mommy!" You must be a terrible person!

Add to this scene the thousands of variables; an alcoholic or emotionally ill mother or father shouting and screaming, beatings, discord. Condemnation for getting to school late, for leaving dirty clothes on the floor, wearing different-colored socks, late for supper, leaving a dirty table . . . "You never do anything right." Oh! For my bottle . . . I've got a thumb . . . or milk and cookies. They will make me feel better!

Middle Childhood

A little girl is playing jacks in the street. The little red ball bounces suddenly out of her reach. It rolls into the gutter and then into the sewer. She cries, she has lost something. An old man comes up to her; he tries to console her. "Here," he says, handing her a lollipop, "everything will be all right, your mommy will get you another one." The lollipop distracts the child. The taste is good. The lost ball has been replaced by the good tasting lollipop. The lollipop "makes everything all right." ("Happiness is a lollipop.")

Mommy had to be away for the whole day, but she promised Tommy she would bring him a present if he were a good boy. Tommy was angry that mommy went away. When she came home that evening, Mommy gave Tommy a chocolate bar and said, "I'm so proud of you. I love you." Those were nice words to hear and it gave good feelings, but the chocolate bar was delicious and its taste soon monopolized the moment. "Mommy loves me, I love mommy, I love chocolate bars." (Chocolate bars are love . . . they make up for the loneliness.)

Nursery school was so much fun with all those kids playing on seesaws, and sliding ponds, and in sandboxes; making Easter Bunny baskets and drawing pictures with pretty crayons, playing with toys and . . . "ring-around-the-rosy, . . . all fall down . . . ouch! . . . that kid hurt me, I'm going to hit him back." The teacher yells, "Harry, stop that! If you don't behave yourself, you're not going to have cookies and milk." "Wow, I'm getting hungry! Besides, the cookies and milk are so good, I better not hit him." (Punishment is *not* having cookies and milk.)

Late Childhood

"I forgot my homework. What's the teacher going to do? It's terrible having to sit here so quiet. I wish I could talk to Sally. Those multiplication tables are so hard. I don't think I'll ever learn them. So many things she's telling me. I don't care about Columbus. Some of these words are easy, but some of the long ones have so many different letters, they're tough! I wish I could go out and play. I wish it were lunchtime, then we could play and we wouldn't have to be so quiet and I wouldn't have to listen to the teacher. I could talk to my friends. I could have something real good to eat." (Eat, and your troubles will fly away.)

"Hey mom, I don't like squash."

"Robert, you should eat it, it's good for you. Besides, you've already had three pieces of white bread with ketchup on it and eaten the meat and potatoes. You should eat more different foods, or you won't grow up to be healthy. Besides, I can't throw out the squash, there are children starving in India."

"It must be terrible to starve, I wouldn't want to live in India. I better eat the squash because they took them away from the starving kids in India." (Eat, it's good for you and your guilt will fly away.)

Later Life

"Let's have breakfast together, so we can relax before you go to work." (Eating relaxes.)

"How about meeting me for dinner, so we can talk." (Eating is communication.)

"Let's celebrate; we will have a special dinner." (Eating is joy.)

"It's your birthday? I should make a cake." (Eating is celebrating.)

"We're going over to their house for the first time. We should bring them a box of candy." (Eating is a gift.)

"What are you going to serve them at the wedding?" (Eating is people and friends and fun.)

"Eat—you'll feel better." (Eating is relief from pain.)

"If you don't cry, I'll buy you a hotdog." (Eating is a reward.)

"I gave her a big box of candy in the shape of a heart for Valentine's Day." (Eating is love.)

"The wine and the wafer are the blood and body of Christ." "Give us this day our daily bread. . . ." (Eating is holy.)

It may seem difficult at first to understand how or why experiences similar to ones I have just shown you leave such a strong, lasting impact on the growing child. If, however, you can imagine for a moment how a child perceives the world in the early years, it becomes clear. Walk up to a child about two years of age, stand next to him, and then look down at him. How very small he is. Now change places in your mind and imagine your parents standing next to you, proportionately as big as you are to that child. They would stand two to three times your height. Their shoulders would touch the ceiling and their heads would reach into the room on the floor above. They would be giants, and this is the way they appeared to you when you were two or three years old. They were your world, your protectors, your source of nourishment, your masters, your gods. Everything they did, or said, was similarly magnified. If they praised you, the praise was powerful. If they condemned you, it was crushing, and if they told you they did not love you, you were unlovable. What they said to you was indelibly marked in your brain, which in those years was fresh and new, and contained relatively little information.

If you were fat as a child and criticized for it, you developed an impaired self-image. You think of your body as ugly and you see others looking at you with anger and ridicule. As you grow into adolescence, these attitudes are strengthened and engraved into the personality structure of your mind. No wonder it is far more difficult to lose weight when obesity begins in childhood. When obesity occurs in later life, it is usually brought about because there is a decrease in activity, but in both the young and the old, food can be a substitute source of comfort, gratification, and satisfaction in a life that is otherwise empty.

THE COLOSSAL CONSPIRACY

The genetic and familial traits we inherit or develop never stop affecting us. Society bombards us with a life style, attitudes, and technology marvelously suited for creating or perpetuating the problem of obesity. It is extremely difficult for anyone to go on a diet, especially when the diet limits not only the *amount* of food that you eat, but the *kind* of food that can be eaten. From dawn to dusk, a barrage of reminders, tempters, and tantalizers permeate all of our senses. The smells from the kitchens of neighboring houses or apartments plague us even though our own kitchen is bare. The wake-up television and radio programs advertise all kinds of goodies. Even our language traps us. Food is identified with all kinds of things. A beautiful girl is "some dish" or a "gorgeous tomato." We'll even refer to a banquet as an orgy. Nationalism has been so intertwined with food, it's surprising we don't salute whenever we hear the words "hotdog and apple pie."

The abundant presence of food and its symbols seem to create an incredible paradox. Its presence is so obvious, we are unaware that we are constantly being sold. It's everywhereness makes it constantly sub-liminal. You might tell your mate, "She's delicious," or "He's so great, I could eat him up," or simply, "Hi, honey." It is even mixed with love and set to music, "You're the cream in my coffee . . ."

Eating can become the substitute for fulfillment in almost every aspect of life. It is something to do when you're bored. It eases the pain when feelings are hurt. It's the only reward left if you didn't get a raise in pay. It may even provide some relief when your sexual needs are frustrated. Thus, food can be the symbolic replacement for all the dep-rivations of life. For some, the increase in body size is identified with power, virility, strength, and protection. Have you ever noticed how many short people are overweight? In others, obesity is a defense mech-anism, an inappropriate excuse for not being active socially or sexually. It may be an expression of anger and hostility, often directed toward self. It can be a means of embarrassing or humiliating others, usually parents or mates. When directed inwardly, it punishes the individual for real or imagined acts and feelings of transgression. It is often an attempt to destroy oneself, when self-image is so low, that the will to live is nonexistent. When directed at others, it substitutes for the inability to express oneself in any other way, because the anger is too intense. Fear of a direct confrontation with resulting harm to others or themselves makes overeating an easier way out . . . so they think.

Eating at night is a frequent problem and may represent a response to various feelings. Nighttime is often associated with loneliness. From early childhood through old age, it is a "dark" time, a time of fear, when help is not readily available and you are left alone with your own thoughts and feelings. It is a time of deserted streets, of shadows, mystery, and death. It is the opposite of the activity, the brightness, the sounds, and the crowds with which daytime is associated. Daytime distractions dis-appear and we are left exposed to the remembrance of life's stressful situations. We may eat to feel secure.

Depression is a disastrous mood for most people. Feelings are dulled and the individual doesn't seem to care about anything. Some people start eating everything and anything they can find. It's as though they were trying to intentionally destroy themselves and everything they have to live for. It has often been said that depression is the other side of anger and depression often represents anger at oneself. Well, how do we solve it? There are two strong forces we can turn to. One force, the instinct for survival, is always there, except in those rare cases where depression is so severe that it leads to suicide. The simple fact that we overeat at a time of depression could indicate that we do care about life and that food represents the baby bottle that will comfort us. The other

factor that we have going for us is our intellect, our thinking and reasoning processes. This becomes a very important part of the Pleasure
Principle and will be referred to again and again. When depression takes
over, positive feeling and thinking disappears and a person's attitude
becomes mostly negative. Some individuals even express depression as
being without feeling at all. It is at this critical moment that the Pleasure
Principle will come to your defense.

The time for decision is nearing. You have been armed with infinite
knowledge of the problem, its component parts and causes. Now is the
final preparation for battle. You must know where you stand. You must
deal with your feelings. You must be motivated and convinced that the
only way to go is down . . . in weight!

Scene 3
The Only Way to Go—Down!

Hunger is not a cause of obesity, what you do about hunger is!

Believe in yourself, and what others think won't disturb you.

Success comes in cans, failure in can'ts.

PREPARING YOUR MIND FOR THE PLEASURE PRINCIPLE

Joe the Glut must be close to fifty now. A few years ago, his mother finally told him the truth about the Polish maid and the stories she used to tell him when he was a child. That night, Joe had some terrible nightmares. He felt the sting of the surgeon's forceps when they removed the buckshot from his buttocks after the hunting accident. He even broke a tooth in his sleep when he dreamt about the encounter with the Kamikaze Karate King that knocked out his front teeth. He finally awoke in a cold sweat as he rewrote the number $265\text{-}\frac{1}{16}$ on the wall of Room 244-B in the State Mental Institution. At 3:00 o'clock in the morning, Joe quietly climbed up to the attic and wiped the dust off an old attaché case lying in the corner. He opened it and gazed at the almost forgotten scale inside. He climbed down the stairs with it and took it out onto the back porch. Joe's family found him sitting out on the back porch as the sun came up. There was a strange knowing smile on Joe's face as the sun began to lighten the land and cast a warm red reflection in Joe's eyes. The sun was rising in Joe's head too; maybe it was just his time of awakening. Maybe, Joe was just entering what they call the male menopause, or climacteric. But, Joe knew what it was, it wasn't just the $100.00 he paid for the package of horse manure, it was all of the events put together which culminated in the final realization brought about by his mother's recent disclosure. Joe finally grew up. He could leave his childhood behind. The magic, myths, and miracles of childhood had made life too painful. He could not live as a child in an adult world, the cost was too great. All of his senses vibrated with the beginning of life. He was in touch with reality and it was invigorating. He took the reins of his life in his two hands, stood up on his feet, took a deep breath, and, with a smile on his face, he started to walk with bold strides. "Joe, that's me, just plain Joe and I am proud of it." The sunrise was beautiful.

You have learned where your feelings came from. Although you may not know specifically why you became fat, at least you have a general idea of the kinds of events that led to overeating as a way of coping. Now it is time to work with those feelings, analyze them and prevent their destructive effect. Like Joe, let us put all the pieces together, take the reins in our hands, use our own two feet and smile . . . the best is yet to come!

FINDING THE REAL YOU

Developing Reality Judgment of Self

Reality Judgment means that you will seek truth on the basis of what is, not what you feel or what you would like something to be. When applied to yourself, it gives you the opportunity to escape from the deceptive feelings and distortions that imprison you. We have been told that it is important to find ourselves. "Once you find yourself, the real you, then everything will be all right!"

What double talk! What nonsense! Where are you supposed to look? Under the rug? On a mountain in Tibet? On Route 66? "Look inside yourself and you will find the answer!"

When you look inside yourself you find out *that you're confused*, and maybe, *why* you're confused. The answer to *who* you are, *what* you are, and *where* you are going, will not be there!

The answers to these questions are self-evident when you analyze the questions.

Who are you? Look in the mirror; that is the physical you. Are you ugly, are you beautiful, or are you somewhere in between? That is a matter of judgment. Who is doing the judging? What criteria are being used? Who asked you? What difference does it make?

Who are you? Who is the personality, the character, the feeling, the thinking, individual you? That's easy! You are everything you have thought, felt, and experienced since you began. You are . . . you! No mystery! No magic! No yolk in an egg waiting for the shell to be cracked!

What are you? A human being! Unique! Similar though, in basic appearance, feelings, and aspirations to the rest of the species. You will probably live to an average age of seventy-two. You are not perfect. Oh yes, you are fat!

Where are you going? You think about that! Head in any direction you would like! But, think it out! No guarantees you'll get there! Make sure you're prepared! Have you got the right equipment? Are you ready for the journey? By the way, the destination is important, but the trip's the thing!

Have I answered the questions?

You're not sure.

Well, let's look at it this way! If *I* answer the questions, it will be my answers for *me*. I'll make some suggestions, I'll give you my arguments for the truth and I'll state the facts as I see them. If they suit you, if they make sense, if you try them on and they feel comfortable, . . . then wear them! We must be the same size! They fit us both! How nice! Let's journey together! Where? The mind, of course!

THE ROAD OF LIFE

The journey we are about to take is along the Road of Life. There are many turns, cut-offs, and alternate routes. The scenery along the route is varied, but, there is always something interesting to see. You must be alert, however, and keep a sharp eye out so that you won't miss a thing. There is another reason for your vigilance: there are pot-holes, washed-out bridges (some you may even have to burn behind you), and barricades. There is occasionally some mud, which can make the going rough. There should also be quite a few surprises. I will give you some technical advice, but you must do the driving. You will have to listen carefully, but to make sure you understand, the important directions and roadsigns will be repeated. Think about them carefully, *analyze* each situation, and don't rush! Then, make your decision based on the reality of your situation. *Treat* each situation on the basis of fact, not wishful thinking! Remember, analyze and treat! I'll be sitting beside you with most of the technical help you will probably need—so use me! Have a good journey! You are the driver, your life is the road.

Self-awareness

Our major concern at the moment is hunger and obesity. These two factors impair our ability to travel and enjoy ourselves. Although we will concentrate on them, the rules will apply to every aspect of our journey. A brief review of how we respond to the road, an awareness of how we move, should help us if we get into trouble along the way. An awareness of the tools we have to correct malfunctions and a knowledge of how to use them will prevent unnecessary delays or failure to complete our trip.

Eating Along the Way

Hunger is basically the feeling we get that says we want to eat something. That feeling can vary in intensity, from just a mild urge to an unstoppable drive. The feeling can be triggered by any one, or all, of our senses. There is even a center in the brain's temporal lobe that appears to direct us in the kind of food we eat. It is responsible for cravings we get for certain foods that contain substances that our bodies require, at a time when the body is deficient in them. The sight of food, or even just seeing something that reminds us of food, can give us that feeling called hunger. Hearing a dinner bell, or for that matter any sound, could trigger the same desire. Our senses of touch and smell, as well as taste itself, can do the same.

It is a common experience with all of us, at work or at play, reading a novel, studying a text, watching television or a movie . . . not hungry in the least . . . when one of our senses picks up a signal and suddenly we feel hungry. How many times has someone said to you, "here, try this," and offered you some kind of food. You refuse . . . but they insist . . . you're not hungry at all . . . you taste it . . . it tastes good . . . now, you want the whole plate! That's a heavy situation (pun intended)! What's happening? What do we do about it?

All of our senses are interconnected through our nervous system, our own private computers, our memory banks, and are interconnected with our bodily functions. In fact, all of the functions of the body, including the involuntary and voluntary activities that it performs, are interrelated. You can even stimulate the flow of saliva in your mouth by just using your imagination. Try it. Imagine yourself sucking on a lemon!

Emotions also are an integral part of this complex system. You might have a need for food, but if you are depressed, you might lose your appetite. Or, conversely, if you are worried, you might develop an appetite when you weren't hungry. In addition, we have all developed habits of eating at certain times. With so many different functions going on at the same time, affected by so many stimuli, it is not difficult to see how easy it is for the sensation of hunger to become confused or tricked into functioning when the need for food does not truly exist. Research done on experimental animals has indicated that the hypothalamus, located in the center of the brain, can be stimulated so as to increase or decrease our appetites regardless of the actual need for food.

Think of it, billions of sensors, nerve pathways, chemical reactions, senses, emotions, habits . . . billions of possibilities of things going wrong . . . Can you beat the system? If so, how can you save yourself? Who or what can stop the villain, obesity? From the caverns of the cranium comes our hero, *the intellect*.

Intellectualize Yourself

It is our intelligence that makes us unique on this earth. If we don't use it, then we are no better than lower animals. If it can get us to the moon, it can get us thin. Our bodies can be controlled. All that is necessary is to be shown the way and then *do it*. Only your intelligence can rule and direct your body and its activities intelligently. It can overrule and restrain, it can change direction. The body will respond to its control. With obesity, it can be comparatively easy, because so much of what we do is only habit. Too much of what we do is done without using our intelligence. It is done either without thinking at all, or by relying upon a portion of our intellect that should have been discarded a long time ago. Our brain stores every experience, every feeling, every thought that we have had from the time it was formed. The feelings and thought processes that were fed into our brains very early in life are still there and under the cover of the experiences, feelings, and thoughts that we've had since. They still direct their primitive responses into our behavior patterns of today. If we, as mature individuals, allow ourselves to behave as we did when we were infants, then we will not survive comfortably in an adult world. The child within us must remain only in memory. Its thoughts were irrational and distorted. It must not be allowed to direct our lives today. *Discard it!*

So, let's use our intelligence, let's use our heads!

Many individuals may still reject the idea that disease can be caused by emotional stress, life's experiences, and inner feelings. You have begun to understand that much of what you feel today, your behavior patterns, responses to life's situations, and personality traits, have their origin in early infancy. They originated in a time and place long since forgotten, so their relationship to the here and now may be obscure or incomprehensible and occasionally even seem absurd and ridiculous.

Well, why is it that you make a vow to lose weight and keep it off, then either never accomplish the goal or, if you do, always gain it back? You make the decision to lose weight and you choose a diet. You stay on it for varying periods of time and then you break the diet. What happened at that moment? Why did it happen? For each of us, the answer to these questions would differ. In my office, most often the reply would be, "I don't know." With a little bit of thought or further prodding, the "I don't know" may change to "I felt like it," "I wanted it," "I had to have it," "I needed it," or "I didn't give a damn." It's at that point that the investigation of the reasons behind the behavior usually stops. Most doctors simply do no have the time for a painstaking investigation into the underlying motivations. But, it is precisely at that point that the investigation should continue. In fact, it is just the beginning. The *why* to all those incomplete answers could be the crack in the door that begins to let in the light. If the answer is an "I don't know," the next question might be, "What did you *feel* at the moment you broke your diet?" If, for example, the answer was "I felt frustrated," it would be important to find out why you felt frustrated. Why did you try to calm the frustration with food? Was it food that you really wanted? Why didn't you use another way to calm the frustration? Did the food make you feel better? For how long? Did the food change the problems that caused the frustration? Was the frustration truly alleviated? If not, then food was not the answer. If the frustration was relieved, why should food have such an effect on a seemingly unrelated problem? Why are food and frustration so closely related? How did they get that way? It didn't just happen!

You now know it was brought about by recurring associations through training and habituation. It was reinforced to the point where frustration was effectively relieved by eating, even though temporarily and inappropriately, regardless of the causes of the frustration. It was a *deceptive* relief of feelings and the effect was, in reality, destructive.

There are other factors you have already learned, so let's answer some of the questions I've asked above.

When you want excess food and you are overweight, the want is for something else, another "need." Your body is already overfed!

The other need is emotional and food will *never* satisfy it! In fact, the other need can never be satisfied!

If a problem causes frustration and it can be solved, then solve the problem. If the problem cannot be corrected, then accept it and divert your thoughts and energies in another constructive, healthy direction. The Pleasure Principle will do the rest.

Self-Emancipation

There is a conspiracy by our culture to shackle us with guilt in every conceivable aspect of living. How many of these situations ring a familiar note for you?

My mother almost died giving birth to me . . . Everything is going so well, something has got to go wrong . . . If I hadn't argued with my father, maybe he would be alive today . . . My parents separated the year after I was born . . . If I don't finish everything on the plate, they'll think I don't like it.

These are just a few of the thousands of guilty feelings that all of us experience each year. Guilt is not all bad. It serves as our social conscience in many situations so that we do not harm ourselves or others. In many instances, however, it is misplaced and unjustified. If guilt is used to channel us into a restricted way of living, or causes us to feel so uncomfortable that it interferes with our functioning in life, then it is unhealthy. If we use the guilt to perpetuate sick, destructive behavior, then we will not be able to change our lives and accomplish healthy goals. In the past when you deviated from your diet and ate something you weren't supposed to, didn't you feel so guilty about the small transgression, that you really went all the way and blew it completely? Instead of just saying "I goofed and I am not going to let that happen again," you made things worse by continuing the uncomfortable feelings. You changed nothing and increased the pain of living. Guilt allows us to avoid the difficult risky path of growth and change in ourselves. By feeling terrible about what we have done, we think we are paying for our sins; in actuality, we punish ourselves more by making the same mistakes over again. If you continue the guilt-ridden behavior of childhood, if you try and place the blame on someone else, you will fail at everything you do, including losing weight and keeping it off. How many times have you abandoned your diet plan when you had an argument with your mate, a problem at work, or faced any disappointing or aggravating situation in life? Shifting the blame didn't help you; in fact, it diverted your attention from your overeating to the anger, frustration, or unhappiness that you were feeling. Only if you grow out of your discomfort, can you find pleasure. To pay penance for your sins is only doubling the punishment. Unfortunately, self-defeating behavior is punishment in itself. The hurt has already occurred, why compound it? What does it serve?

Being fat robs you of a decent quality of life. It is a self-inflicted punishment.

For once in your life, put all the evidence on the table, spend a few good, solid, soul-searching moments. Examine the evidence. What crime have you committed to warrant this punishment? Whom did you kill? What bank did you rob? Are you a child beater, a rapist, or a mercenary? You've been your own prosecutor, judge, and jury. Justify the sentence you have placed on yourself! You can't, and never will, because it is irrational. It is only a distorted, deep, inner feeling. It's a miscarriage of justice. It is cruel and unjust punishment. Your guilt is the only sin!

Inform the judge there is no evidence, there was no crime. The prosecutor was misinformed and coerced. Dismiss the jury! Free the prisoner!

Self-Concept

What is your concept of yourself? In other words, what is your impression of you? How do you feel about yourself? It would be a good idea to sit down and write a description of how you see yourself. The time it will take will be well worth your while. Be completely honest, write down your gut feelings, no matter how good or bad. When you have finished, take each point and justify it. Back up your opinion with facts. Pretend you are an attorney in court and you are presenting your case to a jury. *Feelings* are not allowed unless they can be backed by *facts*.

Naturally, I can't speak for each individual case, but I can make some generalizations that I am sure will apply. Many of the things that you have written down on your list represent feelings, only feelings. When you try to back them up with facts, you are hard put to do so. I am referring to real, hard facts, not silly things like stealing from a 5 and 10 cent store, or remembering the many occasions when you wished your parents would drop dead. On the negative side, if you came up with some terrible things about yourself and you could back them up with facts, these feelings must be resolved. Letting them hang on indefinitely serves no good purpose. Even in our courts of law, a punishment is never indefinite. There is also the possibility that you are unduly hard upon yourself and your "crime" may be exaggerated by your perception of it.

On the positive side of the ledger, you may have found very little to write about. Remember, we are talking about the kind of a person you are, not your accomplishments, although I'll have a few words to say about that later on. You may have left out very important attributes. Let me suggest a few of the things that I think are extremely important.

Perhaps you are kind and considerate. Are you a good listener, sympathetic and understanding? Do you like to love and be loved? Are you sensitive, do you cry at the movies? Do you enjoy a good laugh? Are you a nice person? I am reasonably sure that ninety-nine percent of you cannot justify the negative feelings that you have about yourself, and although there are probably many reasons why you should like yourself, you probably don't. Your early brainwashing has really done its job. If you really liked yourself, you probably wouldn't be fat. Ask yourself, would you injure the health of, or make unattractive, any person, let alone someone you like? Then why hurt yourself?

If you see that you have a lousy opinion of yourself and you cannot justify it, recognize that it is only a feeling and has no basis in fact. What you feel about yourself is therefore a total deception.

Isn't it a common experience in life for an individual to feel inadequate, unattractive, unlovable, or unintelligent in spite of the fact that everyone else says just the opposite? If a thousand people said you were pretty, while you *felt* ordinary, it wouldn't change your feelings. But, if you reasoned it out, thought about it seriously, and worked at it over and over again, then the feelings might change. If the feelings didn't change, you could at least live with them comfortably by *knowing truthfully* that they are inappropriate, irrational, and a ghost out of your past. They can't hurt you unless *you* make them important and meaningful.

You are worthwhile because you are you! No other reason is necessary! Make another list of all the things you must be, do, or have, that you think would make you worthwhile. The Pleasure Principle uses our intelligence to fight obesity.

Are you finished? Okay, now what on that list can you reasonably accomplish? Great, give it a try, don't just talk about it! Now what about the rest of the list, the things you can't reasonably do?

What if a pharmaceutical company offered you a million dollars tax free, if you would lose one pound a week for a whole year? The chances are you would do it. Well, what are your health and your life worth? Could you replace them for any price? Our distortion of values is amazing, especially when it comes to self.

You are worthwhile, important, and significant just because you exist—no justification is needed. The need to hear it from others is a worthless, self-deprecating, self-rejecting state of mind. The unfulfilled emotional needs from your past, which call out through your subconscious to be fulfilled, seek a futile objective and call for a painful waste of time and effort. It is impossible! It cannot be! It must remain unattainable! Discard the voids, the unfulfilled needs, for they existed only for the child. It is over! It is done with! You need no longer attempt to do the impossible by choosing food to replace them. You cannot replace the unreplaceable. If you continue as you have in the past, it is because you choose to do so. You will suffer, because you cannot change yesterday; no one has; no one ever will!

Opinion of self *cannot* be dependent on others. Ask yourself, what it is that you think is healthy or unhealthy about you. On what do you base your values. If you would like to be prettier or more handsome than you are, then ask why it is so important. How would a change in your appearance change your life? Would it *really* change your life? If you think in terms of television stars, movie stars, politicians, or other public figures, how many of them are what you would consider truly "beautiful people"? Not too many! What is beauty? Whose concepts will you accept? Was Lincoln handsome? The beauty we see in Lincoln's face is in the knowledge of what he stood for. Haven't you ever heard men or women talking about someone of the opposite sex who was cute and "oh, so good looking," and then when you saw that individual, wondered why they felt that way? Interest in self, and concern with self will enhance the unique features that you have. Ask yourself what it is that would make you important or worthwhile as a human being. Does there have to be some kind of a monumental achievement in your life, such as finding the cure for cancer, inventing a new source of energy, or solving the world's problems? Did you ever stop to think that if you could just live and let live, and everybody else could do the same, the world would be a far more wonderful place?

If you are fat, however, that is a fact and not a matter of feelings or judgment. It *is* definable and it *is* unhealthy.

We have already seen how obesity can affect one's attitude towards one's self, especially with reference to body image. This poor self-concept often persists even after the individual has lost weight and, in fact, the feeling of being fat may persist even if the patient becomes underweight. Having a healthy self-concept and self-esteem means accepting who you are, but not necessarily what you are. Being fat is not who you are, it is what you are—what you have made yourself.

If you do not like what you are, then you must change it. What does your being fat tell you about yourself? The dislikable things that it tells you are the things that you must change. Only you can change you!

By saying you can't, you have accepted failure.
By saying you can, you risk success.
By saying you will try, you are allowing for failure.

By saying you will, you insure success.
By intending to do, you have destroyed the moment.
By doing, you have made today live.

Self-Criticism

When a relationship breaks up, the first question that individuals usually ask themselves is, "What's the matter with me?", not "What is wrong with the other person?" Perhaps there is nothing wrong with either person. The relationship may have lacked a certain quality that was needed by either one of the parties involved. Those qualities may not even have been healthy ones. So, if a relationship breaks up, it may not be because either party is lacking something good, but might be because one of the parties could be lacking something "bad," some unhealthy quality that is needed by the other.

The opinion of others, whether it be positive or negative, is nothing more than their opinion. It may in no way reflect reality. It often represents their needs, not yours. Their comments, be they good or bad, in no way makes you any different. You are you, and what you feel about yourself will either be healthy or unhealthy.

Not too long ago, I had a woman in my office who was obviously depressed. As she told me her story, it was apparent that I was listening to one of the kindest and most sincere persons I have ever met. I surmised from her story that her boyfriend had a rather unhealthy dependence on his sister. As one might expect, the sister took a dislike to my patient. This sister's great condemnation of my patient was that she "must be a phony because nobody can be that good." I proceeded to tell my patient a story which I hope you will remember many times in your life, if need be.

There was once a bird that sang in the forest and because of the beautiful music that the bird created, the animals in the forest were happy and went about their daily chores with great joy. The wolf was jealous of the bird because of all the love and attention the bird received. One day the wolf called all the animals in the forest together; "We are going to have a singing contest," he said. "The bird and I are going to sing and the one that loses will have his tongue cut out. Porky, I want you to be the judge." Well, Porky the pig was afraid of the wolf, and when the singing was over, he sadly announced that the wolf was the winner. They cut out the bird's tongue and when that happened the forest was a very gloomy place. No longer did the beautiful music of the bird fill the air and all of the animals were sad.

The moral of the story . . . "Never let a pig sit in judgment."
Basic Rule: Judge for yourself.

If you are critical of yourself and the only purpose it serves is to put you down, then you have gained nothing from the criticism. If, however, your self-criticism is used as an opportunity to analyze and change unhealthy behavior, then it is a highly profitable exercise. Criticism offered by others should never be accepted at face value. Weigh it carefully. If you believe it to be just, then start to change that which has been criticized. If you are not sure, talk it over with a professional or a trusted friend. If it is unjust, throw it in the garbage. In truth, criticism should only serve as a positive, constructive force. Remember, consider the criticism, but also consider the source!

Self-Love

When I was a young boy, I was invited to watch the Broadway musical "One Touch of Venus" from backstage, by my cousin who is an actor. As I watched the show, John Boles was about to make his entrance from my side of the stage. He stood right next to me, extremely nervous, wiping the sweat from his brow and then clasping his hands together, as if in prayer. When he exited from the stage, after his opening number, the audience gave him a tremendous ovation. As Mr. Boles reached the wings, again his hands were folded together, he gazed upward and said in a loud whisper, "they loved me, they loved me." I believe I was thirteen years old at the time and I have never forgotten it. I knew even then, at that tender age, that the words, "they love me" were intended to mean the performer and not the performance. It is a wonderful feeling to have others praise your accomplishments, but to need and seek the love of perfect strangers is a tragedy. Love of self and self-worth must come from within. If the meaning of your life is determined by the approval of others, then you cease to exist. The love of a mate, parent, children, or close friends should enrich your life and augment your pleasure. It should never be the fountainhead of your existence. You are the most important person in this world. Who is more important, and by whose opinion? It is necessary and healthy to be self-interested and self-concerned. However, do no confuse it with being selfish. Selfishness is devotion to one's own interest, with carelessness of others. If you are not guilty of being careless of others, then your devotion to your own interest is a healthy self-love. Most of us have been taught that self-interest is wrong. Society teaches sacrifice, putting everything else first, and yourself last. If everyone in the world had a strong devotion to one's own interest, maybe we wouldn't have wars, no one would be willing to die.

Poor self-image comes from being taught not to consider or love self. If a child feels unloved early in life, that feeling can later cause that person to lack self-love. If you feel unloved, you feel you are nothing and if you are nothing, you are incapable of giving love to anyone else. Once again, I ask you to justify any such feeling that you may have with fact. Don't tell me that you haven't got a lover and therefore, you are unlovable. I have two answers for that one. The first is that you may not have met the right person or persons. The second reason is more important: Perhaps your feelings about yourself have kept others from loving you. Perhaps you have made yourself unlovable because of what you feel. Self-love is perhaps one of the most difficult things to accomplish. It pays to give it some thought. Think of someone you have loved. How different are they than you? Were there particular qualities that you loved, or was it because you were expected to love that individual. Do you really think it is some kind of mystical force? If you didn't feel loved as a child, your parents were incapable of giving love. That's how you learned to be incapable of loving yourself.

Not all love for self or for others is necessarily healthy. It may often be the disguise under which we destroy the object of our love. The mythical Narcissus destroyed himself through an all-consuming self-love. The relationship between two people who profess to "love" each other can destroy one or both individuals. One afternoon I treated a woman for a fractured nose, fractured rib, and multiple contusions over her entire body. She admitted that her boyfriend had beaten her up, and that this kind of incident had occurred several times before. When I asked her why she continued to see her young man, she exclaimed, "Because I love him!" I proceeded to tell her a fictional story about another patient I had seen in my office several months before. I described to her almost the exact circumstances she had described to me, and then I asked her what she thought about this other patient's behavior. Her reply was, "Wow, she's a real sicky." I then explained to my patient that I had just told her her own story and that sometimes we see in the behavior of others what we don't see in ourselves. This young woman felt unlovable and proved it by getting involved in situations that would only bring her abuse and hatred. How different is the abuse she received from her boyfriend from the abuse you receive from yourself, or bring upon yourself by being fat?

I am sure that you have all of the attributes of someone who is lovable. If you don't feel that way, we are not dealing with fat, we are dealing only with your feelings. You know where the indefensible, deceptive, irrational feelings belong . . . put them there and please remember to replace the lid, the smell in that garbage can is becoming unbearable.

One area where self-love and sacrifice for others becomes a highly emotionally charged issue is in the matter of parents and children. I once asked a divorced patient "Why don't you make a life for yourself, why don't you try to get a babysitter, or a friend to watch your children, and go out once or twice a week?" She answered, "I didn't want to be selfish." I said to her, "What do you mean by selfish?" She answered, "When you think of yourself." I said, "You're wrong; if you didn't think of yourself, you would cross the street without looking both ways. Is that being selfish? Selfishness is when you never think of anyone else." I suggested that she might split her time, fifty-fifty with her children, or if she felt they needed more time, make it sixty-forty, seventy-thirty or even seventy-five-twenty-five. I explained that it was absolutely necessary that she think of herself and live *her* life; such total sacrifice could only destroy her and her children.

If you have children and hold to the concept that they are the only important part of your life and that you don't count, the results will be a denial of their right to be themselves, to be independent. To better understand this, ask yourself if you would want your parents to live their lives solely for you. Do you want your children to learn to be dependent upon you, to feel obligated, to feel that they do not exist except by your edict, by your help, by your direction? It is only with a healthy attitude of self, that you can give in a healthy way without strings attached, without bitterness, without a need for something in return, without demanding obligations. Sacrifice is rarely necessary. It very often destroys the individuals for whom you are sacrificing, robs them of the opportunity to do for themselves, to be constructive, wholesome, functioning individuals.

Remember that children learn by the example of their parents. Would you want your children to be the self-sacrificing parents to their children that you may have found so tragic in your own parents?

SELF-DETERMINATION AND IMPROVEMENT

Establishing Your Own Standards

Have you ever found yourself thinking that you would like to do something, but then immediately thought, "What will people say?" Who are these people? Who are "they"? When I've asked patients that question, they usually say, "Oh, you know!" and I reply that I don't. When I question further, it usually turns out to be some nondescript segment of the public, maybe the "neighborhood." Most of the time, it's no one who is truly important in the individual's life, or whose opinion should carry any significant weight or authority. What does this kind of thinking truly represent? It's a conditioned feeling brought about by our training and upbringing. It actually represents the thinkings and feelings of our conscience or super-ego. It is the "policeman" or "parent" that we carry around with us in our minds. It serves as our built-in control for behavior that, at times, can be destructive, rather than helpful.

What am I getting at? I am simply asking when your opinion is going to count. When are you going to ask yourself, "What do *I* think about it? What is my opinion? So what if 'they' don't agree. Are 'they' that important in my life? When am *I* going to question the invisible 'they,' and truly make a decision on my own? When am *I* going to recognize that my conscience or super-ego can be wrong? When am *I* going to investigate the truth and logic of the opinions and attitudes that have been programmed into *me* from the day I was born? *When am I truly going to be my own person?"*

Are the standards your own? Why are you accepting the standards of others? By what authority do they set those standards? The ultimate decision is yours anyway. The judgment you hold, whether it is a copy of others or originating from you, is your sole responsibility. You cannot lay off the blame! Thomas Jefferson said, "Your reason is the only oracle given you by heaven, and you are answerable not for the rightness, but the uprightness of your decision." It is rare that anyone else can make a better decision for you than you can for yourself. Set standards of your own!

Being liked for what you are can only happen when you *truly* become your own person. You must exercise your own judgment and accept your *own* worth. Accept yourself and you will be able to accept others. Recognize that what you are is *everything* about you. What you show on the outside does reflect what you feel on the inside. All the rationalization in the world about the motive for dressing sloppily, garishly, or way-out doesn't change the fact that it is truly a reflection of the way one feels about oneself. If you are overweight, the reasons for it may or may not be known, even by you. The opinions that others have about your obesity is not really under your control. There is no question, however, that obesity is unhealthy and must reflect an unhealthy attitude towards yourself.

Let's be practical about it. You say you want to be liked for what you are. But—your obesity is a distorted, unhealthy you. For the sake of argument, we will concede that you are intelligent, loving, witty, kind, understanding . . . a really nice person. Just because you are all those things does not necessarily mean that you will be sexually attractive to someone else. If you are looking for a platonic relationship, then what I have to say here will have no interest for you. However, there are still a thousand other reasons why you should lose weight. For those of you who enjoy your sexuality, remember that getting sexual attention depends upon your ability to use your sexuality to excite others. Sexual arousal is brought about by various stimuli, depending upon the individual. Though someone may love you, it does not follow that because they love you, they must be sexually attracted to you. The fact that you are overweight may very well turn them off sexually. Let's be honest about it, ask yourself, what is so sexually attractive about somebody who is substantially overweight?

Self-determination may not always be a positive force. We may determine the direction of our lives by setting up our own barriers. When we do this, we are determining that we are going to make a turn, and therefore, head in a different direction. More often than not, the barriers are set up unconsciously, without any realization that we are doing it. Obesity is a barrier to achieving a healthy sex life. The sexual problem is usually not a simple one. The possibilities are many. Discovering, understanding, and correcting the difficulties could prove to be extremely difficult and take years of investigation. The rewards, however, are worth it. Not only could you achieve a healthier sex life, but you will probably lose weight in the process. All that you stand to lose is unhappiness, frustration, and weight.

Of the many millions of individuals who are overweight, probably less than one percent can be categorized as *morbidly overweight* (medically significant) and whose obesity is due to a serious emotional illness. If a person is truly convinced that they are not in control of their own behavior, that they cannot do anything about it, then obesity will destroy them because they are defenseless. That individual unquestionably belongs in therapy under the care of a qualified psychotherapist.

For the overwhelming majority of individuals who are overweight, the almost casual statements such as "I can't seem to lose weight" and "I gain, even if I go on a diet!", represent a neurotic escape from responsibility for their own behavior. Remaining obese, for these individuals, represents an excuse to achieve unhealthy needs.

Some people remain fat as an excuse for failure; you can recognize them by such attitudes and statements as:

"I didn't get the job because . . ."
"The boss doesn't like fat people . . ."
"They needed somebody who could wear a size ten . . ."
"I wouldn't look right doing that . . ."

Some remain fat to avoid rejection:

"I won't apply for the job . . ."
"I won't ask her for a date . . ."
"That club isn't for me, because I'm too fat . . ."

Some remain fat to avoid responsibility in their work:

"There is no point in even trying when you're fat . . ."
"I get short of breath whenever I try . . ."
"I can't move as fast as they would like me to . . ."
"I'm too old to lose weight . . ."

Self-Determination

Obesity is not simply a problem of pounds and inches, calories and carbohydrates, food and fats. It is inseparably fused with emotions, feelings, habits, diet, and all of the component parts of an individual's personality. We are what we do, what we say, what we feel, and what we eat. Nothing just *happens*, and there are very few real *accidents* in this world.

Probably the most common excuse given, when an individual has failed at losing weight or keeping it off, is the lack of willpower. Some people use the word and talk about it as if it were some mystical force that you either have or don't have. It is said in such a way that I get the impression most of these patients honestly believe there is some area of the brain that is not functioning or that they are missing this magical ingredient in their psyche. What they are really saying is that they don't want to make choices. They don't want to face reality. They ignore the fact that these choices exist.

If you feel hungry, that hunger must represent one of two possibilities: (1) The hunger is mild and is satisfied by enough food that would allow you to lose weight or at the most, stay the same. (2) The hunger is strong and seemingly drives you to overeat. This is obviously not a physiological message from the body. It is an inappropriate stimulus that in the past brought on an inappropriate response: the destruction of your health.

I think it would be a great idea if we would learn to substitute the words "confronted with a choice" for the word "hungry." Instead of saying "(I have the feeling that) I am hungry," you should be saying, "I am confronted with a choice" (and that decision boils down to) . . . "I'm going to give myself real pleasure" or "I'm going to make myself miserable (deceptive pleasure)."

It is, of course, a matter of exercising one's convictions, doing what one wants to do. The inference is if you don't have willpower, your mind is not your own and you cannot control it. Something, someone, or some force is controlling it for you. Well, that something is your brain. Some of the information it stores from the past is correct, some incorrect, and much of it lacks a key ingredient: *reality judgment.* It is usually the basis for unhealthy and neurotic behavior. The someone controlling your life, then, is *you* . . . the hidden, obscured *you.* Most of the time, you don't realize you are being directed from within or that you *can* control yourself.

Your prime goal should be to develop the key card, *reality judgment,* and feed it into your mental computer enough times so that it becomes a well established habit pattern. It will obliterate the old, unhealthy responses and become a part of your new personality structure. This may not have occurred until now for many reasons. You may have been letting the world run your life out of your past (now internally programmed) and simply did not realize you had to analyze and reinterpret the inappropriate messages from your computer on the basis of up-to-date knowledge and current desires. You had a correction button to push labeled "Reality Judgment" (willpower). All you had to do was push the button enough times, but you didn't. For some of us, the realization that it is simply an unawareness of what willpower really is and that we *can* control it, may be sufficient to effect such control. Unfortunately, this group represents a very small portion of the overweight population.

For the greater majority, the willpower mechanism is intact. It might be a bit rusty, perhaps, but it's still there. The hardware is basically good. Some parts are worn, but they'll serve. There are several steps that you are going to have to take, however, in order to change your programming. First, you are going to have to throw the major switch that determines the *direction* in which you want to go.

For some, the decision to lose weight is not as easy as it once was. You have lost weight so many times and gained it back afterwards that you may have lost heart. You were duped by one fad after another, but now you know there is no magic. You may have had your health jeopardized before, but now you are educated. You fooled yourself into thinking that once you lost weight, you would keep it off forever, now you want a reasonable, sensible, and pleasurable way of doing it. The one thing you have always known, regardless of the method you choose, is . . . there is only one way to go . . . down!

When you have made the *decision* and know where you want to go, you have to *become aware* of the faulty information stored in your brain. Make a note of the most common situation in which the signal of hunger is false and misleading. Whenever that signal appears, push the "reality judgment button" and follow through with your decision. The more you repeat the correction, the weaker the incorrect signals of faulty information become. It takes time and effort, but don't worry; to help you accomplish your task, to fill each day with pleasure, and to make losing weight much easier and even fun, you will have the "Pleasure Principle" (Act III).

How do you push the reality judgment button? Let me show you! (The Pleasure Principle will remind you.) This is very important. You must practice it:

Signal	*(Feeling)* Message from Computer	Button	*(Thinking)* Reality Judgment
	I feel hungry.		My body is overweight, I've already had enough to eat!
	I feel hungry.		I may need something, but I do not need food.
	I feel hungry.		If I eat, I will not be satisfied. I will gain weight and be miserable.
	I feel hungry.		Message incorrect!
	I feel hungry.		So what! I won't starve!
	I feel hungry.		Discontinue message! I'm losing weight! I think I'll go for a walk . . . or read a book . . . or watch television . . . or make love . . . or drink iced tea . . . or I'll call a friend. Reprogramming in process! Reprogramming.

Does this compute? If not, please reread.

If you reason with the impulse enough times, the lack of a response will weaken the force of the message. You will, in effect, create a new conditioned response. The true needs, for example, early infant nurturing and love, *can never be filled*, but they can be understood and accepted. The feelings can be recognized as being from another time and place. Healthy interests and activity can dull the wanting and frustration. However, the best defense against the feelings that have caused you discomfort, confused your needs, impoverished your self-image, and endangered your physical health, is to take the offensive based on a reality judgment of self.

Self-satisfaction

Do you want to change your life? Do you believe losing weight will change your life? What is it that dissatisfies you? More important, what is it that will satisfy you?

Have you ever had the feeling that it's not worth the trouble, or avoided the responsibility of losing weight by saying, "I can't do it" or, "I'm not able to"? You stopped dieting and were left with the hopeless feeling that it was "easier" that way. I am sure many of you fall into this category because statistics and studies have shown this response to be quite common. However, it obviously wasn't the easier way, because if it were, you wouldn't have gone back to dieting so many times. The "Pleasure Principle" will work for you only if you employ it, if you utilize it, and if you pay its salary. For some of you, it may be very difficult, but I assure you it is far *less* painful or difficult than remaining as you are now. If you relinquish the responsibility for what you are, or what you want to be, you are "dead" and cease to exist. Think of all the "rewards" that you have gotten for being the way you are. Does the attention that you get from being fat bring any benefit? Is that kind of attention better than no attention at all? Does it in any way change your life? Does sympathy for your situation really make you feel better?

What is the worst thing that could happen to you if your food intake were limited to an amount equal to or less than what you are burning up? You say you would be hungry; do you mean *really* hungry, starving . . . pain . . . anguish . . . despondency . . . a tearing madness? Or, do you mean . . . "I'm just plain hungry?" Okay, you're just plain hungry, so what? Well, you don't want to be hungry? Okay. If you take in more than what you're burning up, then you are going to be fat! Which will it be, hungry or fat? Your hunger will normalize as you lose weight, gain interests and increase your activity.

Regardless of what causes your obesity, the fact is that only you can change it. Understanding why you are fat can only point out the folly, tragedy, injustice, irrationality, and wrongness of the state you are in. Even if you could place the blame on others, it does not change the fact that only you can create the desired difference in your life. The knowledge of faulty programming, misconstrued messages, reinforced bad habits, deprived basic needs, and unrewarding substitutions will not change what you are, unless you decide to change it. As long as you place the responsibility for your life and what happens to it in the hands of others or by the rules of others, you will remain as your are; you will get worse, suffer, be eternally frustrated, disappointed, and imbued with self-hatred.

This Sunday, why don't you take a stroll through the cemetery; after all, one of those gravestones is going to be yours one day. What are you going to do in the meantime? Are you going to pass up the marvelous opportunity of living? Or will you focus your sights on all the wonderful things that you can do? Do everything and anything you can that will bring satisfaction and pleasure. If it feels good, do it! If it tastes good, eat it—but if you know in your heart that it is only a temporary postponement of the pain that must follow, then *don't* do it. If you made a mistake and it hurt you, then recognize it, and don't make that mistake again. Turn the mistake into a positive experience. Instead of feeling guilty, learn the lesson. If you live to please others, you yourself will become a nonentity; so please yourself and satisfy your own needs. If you wait for others to please you, your life may remain empty and unfulfilled. You may consider others and their opinions, but always judge for yourself. True friends will be happy when you are satisfied and they will admire your self-respect. Lose weight for yourself, and for all of the good things that it will bring you. Losing weight is a challenge to many people, an adventure, and a goal to reach. For you, each day will be an act of living; the loss of weight, an everyday benefit. The progress in losing weight, along with the excitement, the current fulfillment, and the future promise, all act to reinforce the effort and drive. Let each day be a goal in itself. Do not look to the future as the only moment of fulfillment, for when you get there, the drive may be lost, the excitement may disappear and the adventure will be over. Then what? If the expectations were unrealistic, if it was anticipated that all of the problems of life would disappear, and everything would be rosy and wonderful, then there will be a let-down. Frustration and disappointment will set in and the tendency to regain the weight will take over. This is what usually occurs with most diet programs, except for those in which the emotions are dealt with in an intense and serious manner. The "Pleasure Principle" has a built-in mechanism to counteract this kind of effect. If one of your reasons for losing weight is to be healthier or more attractive so that you can find a mate, that is a good reason because it will enhance your life. Finding a *healthy* mate (mentally and physically) should be your goal, not just any mate. Losing weight then becomes an even more logical step. After all, what kind of person wants a fat mate? Is it somebody with good value judgment? Is it someone who admires health rather than sickness? Is it someone who admires a healthy self-concept rather than the lack of esteem? When you are overweight, you ask for less than the best. Your obesity confirms your attitude about yourself. If you choose to lose weight to improve the quality of your life and your health, then you have made yourself important. You have achieved self-satisfaction. Most of the things in life that will bring you satisfaction are well within your grasp. There is only one way to go, the way of healthy self-respect and pleasure. You have been given all of the facts, the pros and cons, *now is the time for decision.*

INTERMISSION

Usher, could you tell me how long the intermission is? . . . Fifteen minutes? . . . I'd like to take a short walk and be able to get back into the theater . . . Thank you very much . . . Oh, hi there! I didn't know you were in the theater. Where are you sitting? . . . Well, what do you think? Pretty heavy, huh? . . . I was going to take a stroll during the intermission, would you like to join me? . . . Well, what do you think? Are you ready for Act III? Well, I'm like you, I'm tired of promises. I've been down this road so many times and ninety-eight percent of them have ended in tragedy. I'd like to see a happy ending for once . . .

Tell me, what about you? Are you going on to Act III? Are you going to lose weight now or are you going to stay fat? The decision can only be yours, you can make it as difficult or as easy as you want it to be. The only real question is, what are you going to do today? Yesterday no longer applies. Tomorrow may never come. What are you going to do today? Are you going to lose weight today or are you going to put it off until the tomorrow that never comes? You can still enjoy your life today, you can improve your life today, you can make a decision for yourself . . . today! Think seriously . . . then decide!

What am I going to do? I'm going on to Act III. I like happy endings!

ACT III
THE PLEASURE PRINCIPLE

*Today is the first day of the rest of your life... Live
it, as though it were your last! ENJOY! ENJOY!*

Scene 1
Pleasure—Real and Deceptive

*We are inclined to see things not as they are, but
as we are.*

If you thumbed through this book while at a bookstore and turned
to this page to find out what the Pleasure Principle is all about, ther
you've short-changed yourself. If you've been reading step by step from
the beginning, you are ready to start enjoying life. Armed with knowledge and understanding, the Pleasure Principle is now yours to put into
practice. The rest of you, please turn to Page One . . .

A tragic beginning doesn't always mean a tragic ending. In both
real life and stories, suffering often gives birth to a new life. Or, as a
psychologist friend of mine once said, "trauma builds character." Well,
it seems that our friend, Joe, finally got some character. It happened a
few years ago when Joe was on a business trip in New York. It was
November as I recall, a November Sunday to be exact. Joe had a few
hours to waste while waiting to go to the airport to catch his plane home.
He decided he would take a walk near Rockefeller Center to see the big
Christmas tree that they erect near the skating rink. It was a rather cold
day and as he was walking back to the hotel, Joe felt the urge we are all
familiar with when our bladders are full. When he got up to the hotel
room, he went to the bathroom and was shocked to find that he was
urinating pure blood. It wasn't painful, but then suddenly, he remembered reading somewhere that painless bleeding from the bladder could
mean cancer. A chill went through Joe's body, a terrible fear gripped
him, and then a strange feeling came over him. He began to feel as
though he was being torn away from the world, as if he was on the

129

outside looking in. As he was riding in the cab to the airport, Joe looked at the skyline of gray buildings, at vague figures walking in the distance, huddled up in their clothing against the cold. Everything seemed so distant now, almost unreal. Even the cab ride didn't seem real. He felt as if he were floating through space with nothing to grab on to, no one to shout to, isolated and alone. He thought to himself, "Oh my God, will this all disappear for me?"

It took only a few days for Joe to have all the necessary tests and then the surgery for a bladder cancer. The surgeon said it was sitting up on a stalk, isolated, and that the chances were great that Joe would not have a recurrence. However, he would have to go for periodic check-ups over the next five to ten years to make sure there would be no recurrence. Joe vowed that he would try to remain acutely aware of each moment of existence. He vowed that each sound, sight, touch, smell, taste, and feeling would be a meaningful and remembered experience. Joe discovered the basis for an exciting, meaningful, and successful way of living which, when applied to your life in general, and specifically applied to your problem of obesity, becomes your foundation for success . . . the PLEASURE PRINCIPLE.

GOING YOUR WAY

Learning the Pleasure Principle is a way of life. It is not some future goal. The only thing that you and I and a two day old baby have in common is today. No one has tomorrow. Losing weight is not something you will accomplish in five months or a year, it is something you can only accomplish today, every day. It is not a goal in the sense of the "end all" or "be all" of living. Your losing weight will be a by-product of the Pleasure Principle in which you learn to live, truly live, and find many things good in each day. If your time is spent in remorse over an unhappy past, then that is the way you will spend today, with remorse. If you deride and abuse yourself over the mistakes of your past, then that is the way you will spend today, abusing yourself. If you feel guilty about your past and think about it and dwell on it, then that is the way you will spend today, feeling guilty. But if you give yourself pleasure, if you seek it in every beam of sunlight and in every shadowed spot, then you will spend your day in pleasure. The quest for pleasure will be an act of pleasure itself. If you seek only pleasure, then how has today been filled? With thoughts and acts and feelings of pleasure. If you see your goal only in the future, then you have spent today without a goal, without an accomplishment, without being. If you worry about tomorrow and what it will bring, then you have spent today with worry. If you live with fear of the future, then you have lived with fear today. However, if you live today with pleasure and if you plan for pleasurable things tomorrow, then your hopes for tomorrow will be a reality, and you will have lived today in comfort and in pleasure.

Say to yourself each morning: "I am the sole judge of my behavior and the only pilot of my life's course. The opinion of others is just that and no more. It is only their opinion. It is my right to accept or reject the suggestions of others. I will do so independently, without obligation or guilt.

"I will serve myself and fulfill my needs only when they are positive, constructive, and healthy. I will serve others and fulfill their needs only when they are positive, constructive, and healthy, and the choice is mine."

You may feel, because of your early teachings, uncomfortable or even guilty at the sound of the word pleasure. Some of you may be ready to throw the label "hedonist" at me. So let me spell it out for you. I believe that the chief good of man lies in the pursuit of pleasure that is healthy, and which protects and holds sacred the rights of all individuals. If you agree with this basic principle, then regardless of your faith, you must believe that all that is pleasurable on earth was created for a positive, good, and healthy reason. The belief that some great power placed this kind of pleasure on earth solely to tempt, trick, or deceive us, would be an unworthy judgment of such a power. It is essential, if you are to live the Pleasure Principle, that you assume the responsibility for your own life, live by your own judgments, and, as Jefferson said, "(you will be) answerable not for the rightness but for the uprightness of your decisions."

With all the tragedy that surrounds our lives not of our own doing, with all of the difficulties and concerns that face us in a modern world, spending all your time seeking pleasure would just about balance the scales. *Stop apologizing for living. Stop apologizing for seeking and enjoying pleasure in life.* To enjoy the miracle of living is the greatest tribute and praise you could pay to any creator. Whatever God you believe in, reflect on the fact that words of praise may nourish the ego of man, but are only platitudes to a God. The act of sanctifying life, making it rich, rewarding, constructive, and healthy, could be the only rational purpose of living. I wonder if you, like so many others, find it difficult to accept pleasure as an experience which is your birthright? Perhaps you are one of those who have often said to themselves . . . "Things are going so well, something has got to go wrong." The feelings of guilt, unworthiness, and uneasiness you may feel whenever you are having a good time, or when something nice has happened to you, are a product of the conspiracy which the unhealthy feelings and ignorance of mankind have passed on to you.

Pleasure is my birthright. Love should be a free spirit, given and received freely. The prerequisite to all love is to love yourself. Consequently, in order to give yourself love freely, it must be without guilt, it must be devoid of the need to be ridiculed, or sacrificed. This is one of the things that occur in many of the diet clubs where the members are publicly ridiculed and where shameful confessionals are given. This too often only feeds the unhealthy needs of the individuals giving those confessions. There is no need to feel guilty, nor feel that you have to pay a penance for being fat. The punishment is built-in, you've paid enough already. Why add additional punishment to it? You've suffered enough because you are fat, so you have to ask yourself, "What crime did I commit that I have to remain in this state of constant punishment and heap insult and injury on top of it?" Declare affirmatively and repeatedly that you will not be a victim of your own misplaced cruelty; "I will not be a victim, I've suffered enough, I haven't done anything to suffer in the first place." Put an end to it. You have done nothing to warrant taking the life of the beautiful person that your are and turning it into a nightmare. Do not restrict yourself from living and enjoying the pleasure of every day.

I am, I count, I have a right to live. You have made the decision to lose weight and the decision to find pleasure in life. Add to this the decision to rid yourself of unpleasant feelings. Ask yourself "What is the worst that can happen?" Usually when you have answered that question honestly, you will find that there is nothing to worry about, nothing to feel uncomfortable about, nothing to even feel unpleasant about. Whatever has happened is over with; it can no longer hurt you unless you allow it. Yesterday should be remembered for two reasons only: To provide you with a pleasant feeling because of a pleasant memory, or as the teaching source of a valuable lesson.

PLEASURE, REAL OR DECEPTIVE?

Once when I was explaining the Pleasure Principle to a patient, I was asked, "If the basic goal is to seek pleasure, then what if your 'pleasure thing' is food, what do you do in that circumstance? What if I want to eat as much of a particular food as I'd like? That question goes to the very core of the Pleasure Principle. Remember, the Pleasure Principle says "being sure it is real and not deceptive." The difference between the Pleasure Principle and all fad diets is that it is based on reality, not on magic, and not on a dream world. It is predicated on what is, rather than on what we would like something to be. Whenever you have over-eaten in the past, whenever you have stuffed yourself, how did you feel about it? Did you feel comfortable? For the few minutes you were eating a particular food, it may have been delicious and you did get some pleasure out of it. The minute you were through, you got up from the table and said, "Oh my god, I did it again," and the pleasure was gone. In its place was misery and other bad feelings. Was the pleasure you had while eating real pleasure? Weren't you, in reality, suspending judg-ment and creating pain and suffering? Weren't the few moments of pleasure actually only a prelude to anguish and grief? Overeating is not pleasure; it is a destructive deception. Now remember, I said overeating, not reasonable amounts of delicious gourmet foods, marvelous hors d'oeuvres, or magnificent desserts. The exquisite taste of mouth-water-ing foods is not deceptive at all. It's like travelling several thousands of miles and spending a small fortune to get a beautiful suntan. If you overdo it, you get a painful sunburn. If someone steals a car for a joy ride, knowing the risk is a year in jail, I think we would all agree, it's a product of unhealthy thinking. It is no different when you overeat. In the Pleasure Principle you are not being denied pleasure, you are being given pleasure. If you choose the deceptive pleasure of overeating, mis-ery follows. Misery breeds frustration and frustration breeds overeating. Interestingly enough, without the Pleasure Principle, the denial of reality pleasure (delicious foods), which is common to all other diets, also breeds misery. Doing without the foods you love follows the same pathway to overeating. Remember, misery breeds frustration and frustration breeds overeating. Therefore, *it is important that you do not deny yourself the good things in life, including the foods you love.*

The Pleasure Principle states that "you should become an expert in your way of life." An expert is a skilled or practiced person. Therefore, our objective with reference to eating, is that you become skilled in the art of eating, a gourmet in the appreciation of food, and have a total awareness of what you are doing. To be practiced means exactly that, to put into effect the Pleasure Principle, to train, practice, and become experienced in its use. Have no fear however, your homework will be pleasurable. Being an expert is more than just doing something as per-fectly as possible. It involves a thorough understanding of food and metabolism, which you now have, and it also requires a direction, which you have already chosen. When we say the word expert, we usually think of the Chris Everts of tennis, the Van Cliburns of music, the Mark Spitzes of swimming, and so on. If you think of them and reflect on what it took to be that kind of expert, you ponder the grueling hours of work and dedication that it took to get there. Most of us are not willing to invest that kind of effort and time into any endeavor. The people who are willing to do that are truly exceptions. Yet, all of us are experts in many aspects of life. The kind of activities I am referring to are those which we do day in and day out, activities that we have become so accustomed to doing that they are accomplished without our even thinking. They are done efficiently, safely and productively. For example, think about driving your car back and forth to work on a daily basis. Most of us, unless we are totally irresponsible, can, and do do it, safely. Think of the many millions of individuals who drive twenty, thirty, or more miles each day from their home to work and back again. While they drive they listen to the radio, think about family and business problems, and generally have their minds on everything except the road. In spite of this, they stop for red lights, slow up for heavy traffic, and turn at the proper times. They arrive at their destination safely and in the shortest period of time, not even remembering how they got there. They are experts at commuting.

If you translate this kind of expertise to another everyday activity, *eating*, you will easily grasp the approach that I am about to present to you. You will learn all the tips, tricks, and techniques required to help you achieve your goal in the easiest, least painful, manner possible. It will be done in such a way that you will enjoy losing weight and benefit from the best things in life as you keep that weight off. Nothing unreasonable is expected of you. There is no dangerous or mythical, magical medicine you must take.

RULES OF THE PLEASURE PRINCIPLE

Losing Weight Permanently
on the Pleasure Principle

There are three rules which *must* be followed in order to be successful at losing weight. These rules are *sacred, inviolate,* and *supreme.* In other words, they cannot, under any circumstances, be broken. It is so essential that these rules be followed, so important that you keep this covenant with yourself, that I have drawn up a contract which you will sign and which will be witnessed by two other individuals. I strongly suggest that one of the other individuals be your family doctor, priest, minister, or rabbi, or any other professional confidant. The other witness should be the second most important person in the world to you (the most important person in the world should be you and you have already signed).

Supreme Rule No. 1

You must eat the foods you love, especially the foods that made you fat.

This rule should raise a thunderous outcry from the purists in nutrition, but I would like to remind my colleagues in the health professions that the purity of their preaching appeals to no one. In spite of the impurity of our ways, our life expectancy is approximately seventy years. Much of the theory and many of the principles of good eating have been discarded and much of what is left is open to serious question. I seem to recall a time when milk, in substantial amounts, was considered a mainstay of a healthy diet. I recall also, how the pendulum has swung in several directions since then. The public is so confused by now that they figure just about everything is going to kill them, so what difference does it make what they eat? If you place a wide variey of foods in front of people, regardless of where they come from, or whether they are slender or fat, the proportion of basic foods they choose will be approximately forty percent carbohydrates, forty percent protein, and twenty percent fat. This proportion remains relatively constant, but the amount of food, that is the total amount of food that the individual takes in, will, of course, vary. The many studies that have confirmed this fact bear out the basic premises upon which the Pleasure Principle is contructed; *we don't eat that badly, we just eat too much!* I believe it is best for patients to seek the kind of diet that they enjoy and that makes them most comfortable. *I do advocate a balanced diet.* That is why I included chapters on food, metabolism, and food fads in this book. I review what my patients have eaten and occasionally have to urge them to balance their intake. The changes required are usually minor. Most of the time you will hear me exclaim, "Great, you had steak, potatoes, and butter this week!" I know it's unorthodox, and I may be the only doctor in the country that would make a statement like that, but there is nothing wrong with steak, potatoes, and butter if they are properly prepared and included in a well-balanced, weight-reducing regimen. What is more important is that the method works. I will also advise my patients that clinical observations have shown that a *moderately* high protein and fat diet meal checks hunger better than most other meals.

The number of meals a day, or the time at which they are eaten, has, in my experience, not proven to be a reliable method of controlling obesity. I leave the meal schedule to my patient's own preference. I believe it is important to think in terms of practicality. Many patients have reported to me that when they tried to eat breakfast, which many authorities believe is the most important meal of the day, the meal stimulated a drive to eat which seemed to continue all day. I think it is much more reasonable to adjust your pattern of eating to your way of life. *Unless a disease process is present,* our bodies appear to be able to handle almost any eating pattern adequately. To place upon yourself an unrealistic expectation, one that you would not be able to fulfill, would be a waste of time. No substantial benefit has ever been proven to warrant altering the pattern of eating, whether it be the number of meals, or the hours of the day at which they are eaten. For some individuals, five or six small meals a day may prove to be the most comfortable and beneficial way for them to eat. For others, one meal a day appears to be most satisfying and ideal for their lifestyle. *Anyone who is suffering from a disease that requires a specific diet is an exception, amd must follow the recommendations of a physician.*

Supreme Rule No. 2

You must write it down before you eat it.

This is the most unbreakable rule of all. I cannot stress its importance enough. There can be *no* excuse for noncompliance. The process of writing down the food you are about to eat, and its value in Pleasure Units next to it, will take no more than a total of five minutes a day. It can be done anywhere, anytime, in any shape, manner, or form. It might be preferable to write it down in a small notebook, but it isn't necessary. It won't make any difference if you write it on a piece of toilet paper, gum wrapper, matchbook cover, or the bottom of your shoe. You can write it in pen, pencil, burnt matches, grape jelly, or even lipstick, as long as you write it down. *It must be done!* What possible excuse could there be for not doing it? Many of you have to sign in at work when you go to your job. You have to stop at red lights when you drive your car. You have to put on clothes when you walk out the door. You have to obey a thousand and one rules each day. Here is one rule, which if kept, will lift many other restrictions in your life (those placed on you by your obesity). Five minutes of your time invested in writing a few words and a few numbers and, in return, you can eat whatever you like to eat, lose weight, and keep it off . . . permanently. Look at the trade-off; one minor inconvenience for a thousand benefits that spell out pleasure and health in your life. *There can be no excuse.* If you do not do it, it simply proves that your desire to lose weight is self-deception.

I am sure that many of you know of someone who has looked or have had the experience yourself of looking, at the scale at the end of a week of trying to lose weight, and seeing that your weight has remained the same. In some instances, you may even have gained weight. During the many years that I have practiced, it was such a common experience that I developed a little technique to help patients become aware of what has occurred. When they get that rare disease called "how come I gained weight when I ate nothing?," I answer them, "I don't know, but I want to find out as much as you do why this very unusual thing has occurred." I suggest that we do a simple scientific investigation ourselves. I tell them that during the next week they should write down everything that they put in their mouths. I even suggest that if they bite off a fingernail and swallow it, they should list that. I ask them to look up the value of the food they are eating, on the Pleasure Unit list, and to bring it back with them when they return the following week. I explain that when I see what they have been eating, I can discover what is wrong. Then, I will be able to decide whether it is necessary to proceed with very expensive tests involving the glandular system. Ninety-nine times out of a hundred, when patients return the following week, they have lost weight!

Recently, a seventy-five-year-old patient decided to go on the Pleasure Principle Diet. When he returned at the end of two weeks, he had lost six pounds. During our discussion, he agreed, as do most patients, that it was easy, enjoyable, and gratifying. He made one comment I felt was so important that I jotted it down. It summarizes the essence of Supreme Rule No. 2. He said, *"When you write it down, you look at it differently."* Almost all forms of psychotherapy, regardless of their theoretical approach, seek to accomplish one common goal; that goal is probably best described in one word, "awareness." *When you write it down, you look at it differently . . . you become aware!* The Pleasure Principle is not just a way of losing weight, it is a way of life. If you are to seek pleasure in everything you do, awareness is essential. You cannot lose weight permanently without it.

I mentioned that you must write the food down that you are going to eat, along with its value next to it. I call the value a *Pleasure Unit.* The Pleasure Unit is a proportionate value given to food that is extremely easy to remember. In the chapter on Pleasure Units, you will find an exciting, unique concept that allows you to assign a value to any food *without* having to carry around a scale or a ruler. It will facilitate your becoming an expert in the foods you love to eat.

Supreme Rule No. 3

Lose weight at a comfortable and pleasurable rate.

The rate at which you lose weight is determined by the number of Pleasure Units you spend on food each day. The number of Pleasure Units you spend is completely up to you. I will, however, give you some guidelines to ensure success. The more Pleasure Units that a patient spends while losing weight, the slower the weight loss. The fewer Pleasure Units spent, the faster the weight loss. The average number of Pleasure Units that can be spent on food while still ensuring weight-loss is between 1,000 and 1,500 Pleasure Units a day. If you spend only 1,000 Pleasure Units a day, you will lose weight at your body's optimum rate. If you spend 1,500 Pleasure Units a day, you will still reap pleasure by losing weight, but less quickly. If the number of Pleasure Units spent goes beyond the number that the individual can consume by their daily activities each day, then your Pleasure Units become "misery units." The choice is yours. I promised at the beginning of the book that there would be two words that I would not use in *The Pleasure Principle Diet*. So instead of saying the word, I am going to spell it out for you in the next sentence. At this point, I am sure some of you are saying that Pleasure Units are C-A-L-O-R-I-E-S. *Pleasure Units are not C-A-L-O-R-I-E-S*. Pleasure Units bear a resemblance to that word, but they definitely are not, and when you get to the Pleasure Unit chapter you will understand more clearly why that is so.

A rapid weight loss can be deceptive. It is more likely to represent a loss of lean tissue rather than fat. The Pleasure Principle is not a crash program in which you severely restrict your intake. If you go below 1,000 units a day, you can very quickly dehydrate the fat in your tissue. Dehydrating means you pull the water out of the tissue fat. This water then goes into the general circulation and passes out of the body as urine. You will lose weight, as shown on the scale, because of the excretion of this fluid. The fat itself, however, has hardly been touched at all and your body is converted to a "dried-up sponge." When you return to healthy eating, the water is quickly reabsorbed by the body to rehydrate the fat and you suddenly gain back a good portion of the weight that you lost. If your intake is below 1,000 Pleasure Units a day, it becomes more difficult to eat a balanced diet. Without a balanced diet, you jeopardize your health. The limit of 1,000 to 1,500 Pleasure Units is not a hard and fast rule. There are some exceptions, and they have to do with age, height, and body frame. These exceptions will be explained for you in the chapter on Pleasure Units. Some deviations can be tolerated to a limited degree as long as it is not an "everyday affair" or for more than just a few days. I don't really care what you eat. If you want to use your Pleasure Units on nothing but ice cream all day, be my guest. I don't advocate it, and it is obvious that it resembles the "fad" approach. However, if you did want to do it for a few days, go ahead. The chances are you are not going to do it everyday. I have great faith in people and I don't honestly believe that there are that many bad or unknowledgeable eaters in this country. There is no strong evidence that a few days of unreasonable eating, or even fasting, does any measurable harm. It is obviously something that should be avoided in individuals who are under a doctor's care for a specific disease. The rate at which you wish to lose weight is a matter of free choice and can vary from day to day or week to week. Why must you lose weight yesterday? It took you a long time to get where you are and, like most things done in haste, if you lose it quickly, the results are not attractive. The effect can be unpleasant and the stress can be great. Everyone's needs are different, and it pays to think carefully about what pace of weight loss would suit you best. Some individuals have been battling the problem of weight for a long time. The ability to fight that "inner drive" to overeat has been seriously undermined. For these individuals it would make sense to start slowly, to allow themselves as many Pleasure Units as possible, even though the weight loss would be much slower. Some people never seem to learn. It is usually the individual who is markedly overweight that tries to lose it the fastest. They are the ones that use the "crash-method," and that has to be the worst way to approach the serious long-term weight problem. Remember, it definitely makes sense to learn to crawl before you learn to walk, and to be able to walk before you can run. Experience has taught me that it is easier to get people to maintain a reasonable intake than it is to ask them to go to extremes. Moderation, obviously, becomes the key note and pleasure is more likely to be achieved through moderation. If you lose weight rapidly, it may not allow for an emotional adjustment to your physical change. When individuals drastically reduce their food intake, their new life style tends to isolate them from the mainstream of society. The Pleasure Principle is designed to make the reducing effort minimal and enjoyable. If you are expecting that the loss of weight alone will change your whole life, you are expecting the impossible. Losing weight will improve your physical appearance and health, but the change in self that is absolutely necessary to create a better quality of life may require more than the Pleasure Principle. The Pleasure Principle places you first, but you must be willing to do the same. Though you may have had problems with your family because of your weight, these problems could get worse once you have reduced. In this instance, professional help can mean the difference between success and failure. Though you lose weight and become slender, you may have to learn, or relearn, thinking like a thin person. Discussions with a mental health professional can help you develop an objective evaluation of your situation and give you the strength and vision to create a healthy, new, *pleasurable* life.

The price that we pay for following this program is far less than the price we pay when we continue in a state of unhealthy obesity. *You must not break the Three Supreme Rules.* It will take effort on your part, but that effort will be minimal. I believe you will find these rules much easier to follow than the fifty-five mile speed limit. If you look upon this program as a trip through life, then the rules are basically simple. You can travel anywhere you want to; you can eat anything you want to. You have a speed limit, but it is reasonable. The limits on Pleasure Units are likewise reasonable. You must know how to drive and it must become second nature to you. You must be a gourmet, and also an expert on the *value* of the foods you eat. You must be familiar with the causes of "accidents" (straying off the diet). When you accept the dangers as real, and not to be ignored, then you will travel safely and the trip will be pleasurable. It is a great feeling to be able to say to yourself, "I can eat anything I want, I'm no different from everyone else, and I'm controlling my weight like an expert. What I am doing is for my body, my life, and my future." You no longer live in a fantasy world. The old adage, "What you don't know doesn't hurt you," is changed to "What you do know won't hurt you." When you write down what you are going to eat and see what you are doing, you have called your intelligence into play. It is your greatest defense against neurotic behavior. When you see what you have eaten for the day, you may realize that you have created your own fad diet (which you can add to my list in this book). With the knowledge you have gained, the chances are you will correct this unhealthy state of affairs easily, with only a few alterations. When you choose and vary your own rate of weight-loss and let it fluctuate with the needs and healthy feelings of each day, you have finally taken a major step in running your own life.

A universal experience for an individual starting a weight reduction program is a rapid loss of weight the first week or two, and then a marked slowing down. Why does this happen? During the early period of dieting, water and protein are lost along with the fat that is being metabolized. Extra weight is, therefore, lost, but only a portion of it is fat. As the size of the fat cell is reduced, it becomes more difficult to extract the fat from the cell, hence, you lose weight at a slower pace. However, if you keep in mind that the weight loss is proportional to your total body weight, you won't feel cheated. For example, a patient who wants to lose

150 pounds would, if he lost 15 pounds, lose ten percent of the undesirable weight. A patient who is only fifty pounds overweight would be doing equally well by losing five pounds, as this would represent ten percent of the weight that has to be lost. Whatever you do, don't compare yourself with someone else, unless you do it on the basis of percentages. If you must, at least do it on a proportional basis. It is important that you abandon the irrational, frantic idea that your weight has to be lost by tomorrow. Remember, this time you truly have an opportunity to lose weight *permanently*. The results of your labor, as well as your enjoyment and fun, will not be measured on the scale alone. You will see it in the mirror. You will feel it in your available energy. You will measure it by your beltline. You will know it in your mind and heart because it is a product of your way of life. You have done your thing!

THE PLEASURE PRINCIPLE CONTRACT

From this moment forward I pledge that:

I will seek real pleasure in every moment of my life.
I will make my own decisions and take total responsibility for them.
I will improve and maintain my health.
I will lose weight at a safe and comfortable rate.
I will eat the foods I love without guilt.
I will write down everything I intend to eat before I eat it, and place the number of Pleasure Units next to it.

Witnesses:

_____

(Very important person in my life)   (Signed)

_____

(Doctor or Clergyman)

Dated:

_____

Where signed:

_____

Scene 2
Pleasure Units—Limited, Unlimited, Self-Limited

When you write it down,
you look at it differently!

Would you drive your car down a city street at a speed of 100 miles per hour? The answers to that question might be: "What do you think I am, crazy?" "You can get killed that way." "Of course not, I would end up in jail. I'm liable to kill someone." "You should know better than to ask a question like that."

Would you jump off a twenty-story building, flap your arms and expect to fly? The answers to that question might be: "Would you?" "What a dumb question!" "Ah, come on, be serious." "Either ask an intelligent question or stop wasting my time."

The two questions seem absurd, ridiculous. Everybody knows what the answers are. Nobody in his right mind would try either stunt. Yet when I ask the next question, which is equally absurd, practically everyone who is reading this book has done it.

Would you take in more energy than your body is burning up and expect to maintain or lose weight? The answer is simply "NO!"

Why is it that you have never done the things mentioned in the first two questions, but for years have done the third? Is it because you believe the consequences from the first two acts are worse than the result of the third? We have seen that this isn't true. Is it because the consequences of the first two acts are imminent, and you believe that the consequences of the third act aren't? That is not true either. You *will* gain the weight *immediately*. Maybe it's because you don't really know when you overeat, or how much you overeat. I constantly hear people say: "I don't eat that much." "One more piece can't make any difference." "It's not that fattening." "How much can there be in that little piece of candy?"

If you knew how much energy was available in everything you ate, and if you knew how much energy you burned up each day, would you then knowingly put on more weight?

Absolute Fact. If you take in more energy than you burn up, you will gain weight.

Absolute Fact. If you want to lose weight, you must take in less energy than you burn up.

It is not difficult to figure out that the only way you can lose weight is to take in less energy, burn up more, or both. In order to do this, you must know what you are doing and keep track of it. Counting c-a-l-o-r-i-e-s has not worked because it is cumbersome, difficult to remember, and requires special measuring devices. If you have ever looked at some of those little books with the long list of foods, it becomes very discouraging because they are impossible to use on an everyday basis. For some items on the list, it is not too difficult because they measure the foods in teaspoons, tablespoons, glasses, or cups. It *is* discouraging when they use the following descriptions: "Three ounces, one-half pound, two and three-eighths inches in diameter, three inches by two and one-half inches, one piece in a two-pound jar, average serving, or usual portion." It's bad enough that you have to look up something every time you want to eat, but if you have to walk around with a scale and a ruler, that does it!

The concept of Pleasure Units provides an easy, simplified way of estimating the relative values of foods and remembering them. The method is quickly learned and no special measuring devices are necessary. There will be nothing to weigh and nothing to measure.

The Pleasure Principle is unlike any method of losing weight that you have used before. You will have to abandon the idea that there are restrictions on the kinds of foods you can eat. So there is no misunderstanding, I am going to list a few basic rules you must not forget.

Do not use gimmick foods such as dietetic desserts and protein drinks. After all, if you go to a club or a restaurant, or if you are visiting friends, these are not what you will be served. You are not learning to be a "food freak" or a social outcast, but are learning to use normal foods.

Eat any food you like, usually the foods that you have been eating most of your life and will probably continue to eat the rest of your life. Eat anything you want, but in moderation. The moderation I speak of

will not be left to guesswork. You can use diet soft drinks if you want
to and if you like them. Their use is so widespread they can be considered
normal.

> Do not deprive yourself of anything.
> There is no food that is excluded.
> There is no food that is forbidden.
> Any food you want to eat is okay! Fine! Wonderful! Permitted! Allowed!
> Do you get the message?

I insist that you eat what everyone else eats while you are losing
weight. If you follow the methods as outlined, you will not stand out
like a sore thumb in public. You will be able to go to parties, vacation
in Europe, go on cruises, and eat out with friends in complete comfort.
You must abandon all feelings of guilt when you have an ice cream soda,
a piece of chocolate cake, or a whipped cream pie. Because you have
allowed for it, you are entitled to it. Enjoy it; you deserve it!

THE PLEASURE UNIT

The Pleasure Unit is a proportional estimate of energy value in
foods. The Pleasure Unit list contains the most frequently-eaten foods.
All foods will be listed with an energy value of twenty-five or multiples
of twenty-five; for example:

Food	Amount	Pleasure Unit
Marshmallows	1	25
Appetizers, miniature	each one	50
Breads	1 slice	75
Cereals	1 cup	125
Cereal, cooked	1 cup	150

There are just a few exceptions you may encounter in the list. There
will be a few items that are listed with Pleasure Units of five, ten, and
fifteen, but they will be easy to remember, especially if you eat them
frequently and are following the supreme rules which are printed at the
top of every page.

Estimating Pleasure Units

I said that you would not need a scale, ruler, or any special measuring device. All of the things that you will need to estimate the Pleasure
Units in food will be with you at all times. A teaspoon, a tablespoon, a
glass, and a cup are common items on every table. If not, which would
be a rare exception, you can estimate. Where it says a cup, it does not

mean a measuring cup. It means a standard household teacup, the kind found in every cupboard. When the list indicates a slice, it refers to a standard slice, such as you will find in a loaf of bread or in packaged cheese. Where the words "Pleasure Portion" (abbreviated PP) are used, it means a piece of food, one-quarter-inch thick (which you can estimate), the size of the palm of your hand. The palm of your hand should be represented by an imaginary circle; the circle's diameter extends from the base of your fingers to the beginning of your wrist.

For a slice of chicken, for example, the Pleasure Portion size would be 100 Pleasure Units. If you are a woman standing five feet tall, don't feel cheated when you compare the palm of your hand with that of your boyfriend who happens to be a football player and is six feet, four inches and weighs 280 pounds. You never ate as much as he did in the first place; in fact, you probably couldn't eat as much as he does if you tried to.

Ninety-nine percent of the people eat between fifty and seventy-five different foods. Therefore, the most you will have to learn is the value of seventy-five items. However, it should be far less than that. If you will notice from the list above, in which I gave you examples of foods, all dry cereals were listed together. If you ate several kinds of dry cereals, you would have to memorize only one value for all of them. It is for this reason that the Pleasure Unit List is a lot shorter than any other list that you have seen. It will take very little time and effort to write down everything you put in your mouth . . . about five minutes a

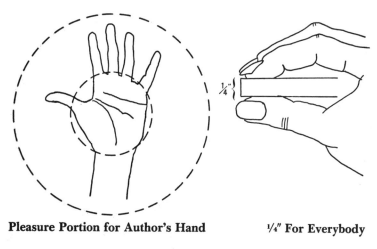

Pleasure Portion for Author's Hand   ¼″ **For Everybody**

Figure 1

day! If you don't keep an accurate account of it, your *stomach* will do it for you. Even a piece of chewing gum must be counted. Remember, if you list a piece of toast, don't forget to put the butter or the jam down also. When you are having dry cereal, and then add milk and sugar, you must add them to your count. When you have an egg that is boiled or poached, it is just an egg. However, if you scramble the egg in a pan with butter or margarine, the butter or margarine must be added to your total.

It is impossible to list all foods; however, I will give you a few helpful hints to show how you can closely estimate the value of almost any dish put in front of you. For example:

1. Anytime you bread a portion of food the size of the palm of your hand, you add fifty units. (Example: Breaded veal)
2. Anytime you fry a portion the size of the palm of your hand, you add fifty units. (Example: Pan-fried steak)
3. One tablespoon of thin sauce or dressing is twenty-five units.
4. One tablespoon of thick sauce or dressing is 50 units.

If you were to have chicken parmigiana and it's not listed, you could easily add up the ingredients based on a portion of chicken the size of the palm of your hand and end up with the following:

Food	Pleasure Portion	Pleasure Units
Chicken	1	100
Breading		50
Frying		50
Cheese	1 slice	100
Sauce	2 Tbs.	100
	Total	400

There you have it, quickly and easily, chicken parmigiana.

You will be able to see a similarity between certain types of vegetables, cereals, sauces, etc., that groups them together by units. If you go on a trip through Europe or Asia and you sit down to unfamiliar dishes, you can compare a strange, leafy vegetable with spinach, or an unusual bean with our baked beans, and so on.

The Pleasure Principle offers you the ultimate freedom while losing weight. You are not only free to choose the foods you'd like to eat, but you can increase the number of Pleasure Units each day that you can spend on food by earning Pleasure Credits. The number of Pleasure Units you spend each day is limited to between 1000 and 1500 units, depending upon how fast you want to lose the weight. However, you could still lose weight at the same rate or faster and yet eat more food. You will find out in the Scene, Pleasure Begets Pleasure, that you can earn an almost unlimited number of pleasure credits which can be spent on food if you so choose. In this way, the management of Pleasure Units is completely under your control. They are self-limited, and therefore can be manipulated to provide you with the most pleasure possible.

LIST OF PLEASURE UNITS
FOR COMMONLY USED FOODS

Food	Amount	Pleasure Units
A		
A-1 Sauce	1 t.	10
Abalone	PP	100
ALCOHOLIC BEVERAGES		
Ale, Beer, Malt	1 gl.	100
Cocktail	4 oz.	150
Grog	1 c.	200
Highball	1 gl.	150
Liqueur and Brandies	1 oz.	100
Whiskey	1½ oz.	100
Wine, Champagne		
Dry	4 oz.	75
Medium	4 oz.	125
Sweet	4 oz.	175
Mixed Drinks with cream	1 gl.	225
Almonds	1	10
Ambrosia	1 c	150
Anchovies	1	10
Anchovy Paste	1T.	50
Apple	1 sm.	75
Apple, baked with sugar	1 sm.	200
Apple Brown Betty	1 c.	400
Apple Cider, hard	1 c.	100
Apple Butter	1T.	50
Apple Sauce	1 c.	100
sweetened	1 c.	200
Apricots, fresh	1	20
canned	1 c.	200
Apricot Butter Preserves	1 T.	50
Apricots, dried	1	15
Artichoke	1	75
Artichoke Hearts	1	50
Asparagus	1	5
Asparagus Tips (canned)	1	5
Avocado	1 sm.	400
B		
Bacon	1 strip	50
Bacon, Canadian	1 sl.	50

Food	*Amount*	*Pleasure Units*
Bagel	1	175
Baked Alaska	1 c.	350
Baked Beans	1 c.	250
pork or molasses	1 c.	350
Banana	1	100
sliced	1 c.	125
Barbecued Beef	PP	150
Barbecued Chicken	PP	150
Barbecue Sauce	1 T.	50
Barley (cooked)	1 c.	200
Bean Sprouts	1 c.	25
Beef, boiled	PP	125
Beef, creamed	1 c.	300
Beef, curried	1 c.	300
Beef Stroganoff	1 c.	300
Beef Steak & Kidney Pie	1 c.	300
Beef Stew	1 c.	200
Beet Greens	1 c.	50
BEVERAGES, COMMON		
Carbonated (soda)	1 gl.	100
Cider	1 gl.	200
Coffee	1 c.	0
Eggnog	1 gl.	300
Fruit Drinks	1 gl.	100
Fruit Juice	1 sm. gl.	100
(except prune,	1 sm. gl.	125
tomato)	1 sm. gl.	25
Ice Cream Soda	1 gl.	275
Milk	1 gl.	150
(chocolate)	1 gl.	200
cocoa	1 c.	175
cocomalt	1 gl.	275
coconut	1 gl.	250
shake	1 gl.	500
skim (low fat)	1 gl.	100
Ovaltine	1 gl.	225
Tea	1 c.	0
Biscuits	1	75
Blackberries (canned, syrup)	1 c.	200
Black-eyed peas (canned, drain)	1 c.	200
Black Walnuts	1	25
Blintzes, cheese	1	175
fruit	1	100
Blueberries	1 c.	100
Blueberry Muffin	1	150

Food	Amount	Pleasure Units
Bleu Cheese	1 T.	75
Borscht, beet	1 c.	75
Bouillabaisse	soup plate	500
Brains	1 c.	200
Bran Muffin	1	100
Brazil Nuts	1	25
Bread	1 sl.	75
Bread Crumbs and Stuffing Mix	1 T.	25
Breadsticks	1	50
Broccoli	1 c.	50
Brown Bread (Boston)	5 PP	75
Brussels Sprouts	1 c.	75
Butter	1 pat	50
	1 T.	100
Butter Cookies	1	25
Butter Crackers	1	25
Butter Frosting (any flavor)	1 T.	50
Butternuts	1	25
Butterscotch Sauce	1 T.	25

C

Food	Amount	Pleasure Units
Canned Beets	1 c.	50
Cabbage, boiled	1 c.	50
raw	1 c.	50
stuffed	1	150

CAKES (with nuts, add 50, with icing, add 50)

Food	Amount	Pleasure Units
Angel Food	TPP	150
Cheese	TPP	350
Chocolate	TPP	250
Coconut	TPP	300
Coffee	SPP	100
Crumb	SPP	100
Cupcake	1	100
Devil's Food	½″ sl.	275
Eclair	1	275
Honey	½″ sl.	150
Jelly Roll	½″ sl.	200
Marble	½″ sl.	125
Pound	½″ sl.	125
Sponge	½″ sl.	125
Strawberry Shortcake	TPP	350
Strudel	1	225
Upside Down	SPP	275
Whipped Cream	TPP	350
All other cakes	TPP	200
with icing add		50

Food	Amount	Pleasure Units
CANDY		
All chocolate or chocolate covered candy bars	1	300
Bon Bons (chocolate creams, fruits, nuts, etc.)	1	50
Candied Fruit	1	100
Candy Apple	1	275
Caramel	1	50
Fudge	1	100
Gumdrop	1	15
Hard Candy (small Life Savers, squares, etc.)	1	10
Jelly Beans	1	10
Kisses, Choc.	1	25
Lollipop	1	100
Marshmallow	1	25
Mints	1	10
chocolate-covered	1	50
Peanut Butter	SPP	100
Cantaloupe	½	50
Capon, roasted	½	225
Catsup	1 T.	25
Caviar	1 T.	50
Cereals, cold	1 c.	125
cooked	1 c.	150
Cinnamon Toast	1 sl.	100
Celery	1 stk.	5
cooked	1 c.	25
CHEESE		
All	1 sl. or 1 oz.	100
Creamed Cottage Cheese	1 c.	250
Cream Cheese,	1 T.	50
whipped	1 T.	25
American, grated	1 T.	25
Cheese Spreads	1 T.	50
Farmer Cheese	1 c.	400
Pot Cheese	1 c.	400
Cheese Blintzes	1	175
Cheese Soufflé	1 c.	200
Cherries	1	5
Chestnuts (roasted)	1	5
Chewing Gum	1 stick	5
Chicken	½ sm. or PP	100
Chicken à la King	1 c.	750
Chicken Cacciatore	PP	400
Chicken Chop Suey	1 c.	550

Food	*Amount*	*Pleasure Units*
Chicken Chow Mein	1 c.	250
Chicken Fat	1 t.	50
Chicken Fricassee	1 c.	225
Chicken (fried)	½	325
Chicken Livers	1	50
chopped	1 T.	125
Chicken Pot Pie	1 c.	500
Chicken Salad	1 scoop	225
Chili Con Carne	1 c.	500
with beans	1 c.	350
Chipped Beef	1 c.	175
Chips, Crisps, and similar snacks	1	15
Chocolate Milk	1 gl.	200
Chocolate Pudding	1 c.	500
Chop Suey, pork	1 c.	600
Chopped Steak	¼ lb.	350
Chow Mein, pork	1 c.	250
Chuck Steak (with bone)	PP	100
Chutney	1 t.	25
Cinnamon		0
Cinnamon Bun	1	100
Cinnamon Muffin	1	100
Clams	1	10
Clam Broth	1 c.	50
Clam Chowder	1 bowl	275
Clam Juice	1 gl.	50
Clams, stuffed, deviled	1	20
Clams, fried	1	25
Cobbler, Apple	1	300
Cocoa	1 c.	125
with milk	1 c.	250
Coconut		
milk	1 c.	600
water	1 c.	50
shredded	1 c.	450
cream	1 c.	800
Codfish	PP	100
Codfish balls	1	100
Coffee, black	1 c.	0
Cola	1 gl.	100
Cole Slaw	1 c.	25
Compote, Apricot-Apple	1 c.	100
COOKIES		
Animal Cracker	1	15
Chocolate Chip	1 med.	50
	1 lg.	75

Food	Amount	Pleasure Units
Oreo	1 lg.	50
All others	1	50
Corn, fresh frozen	1 c.	150
Corn Fritters	1	175
Corn, canned	1 c.	150
Corn grits	1 c.	125
Corn on the cob	1	100
Corned Beef	PP	200
Corned Beef Hash	1 c.	350
Crab Apples	1	50
Crab, deviled	1	200
Crabmeat	1 c.	125
cocktail	1 c.	200
Crab, soft shelled	1	100
CRACKERS		
Cheese	1	15
Cheese Sandwich	1	50
Graham Cracker	1	25
Matzos	1 sheet	125
Melba Toast	1 piece	15
Soda Cracker	1	15
Thin Cracker	1	10
Tidbits, oyster	10	25
Cranberries	1 c.	50
sauce	1 T.	50
CREAM		
Half and Half	1 T.	25
Non-dairy (dry)	1 t.	10
Whipped, heavy	1 T.	50
Cream Puff	1	175
Cream Sauce	1 T.	25
Croutons	1	5
Crullers	1	150
Cucumbers	1	25
Crepes Suzette	1	225
D		
Danish Pastry	1	225
Dates	1	25
Date Nut Bread	1 sl.	100
Dates, stuffed	1	50
DINNERS		
Frozen	1	400
with sauce	1	500
with dessert	1	600
Dips	1 T.	50
Doughnuts	1	150

Food	Amount	Pleasure Units
French	1	200
Jelly	1	250
Sugared	1	175
Dressings		
French	1 T.	100
Oil & Vinegar	1 T.	50
Roquefort cheese	1 T.	125
Russian	1 T.	50
Duck	½	300
with dressing	½	375
Dumplings, apple	1	75
E		
Eclair	1	275
Eggs	1	75
fried	1	100
Eggs Creole	2	175
deviled	1	125
Egg Cream, chocolate	1 gl.	300
Egg Foo Young, Chicken	PP	250
with pork	PP	350
Eggnog (brandy)	1 c.	300
Eggplant	1	50
Baked-Italian	PP	350
parmigiana	PP	400
Egg Roll (Chinese)	1	175
Enchiladas	1	200
English Muffin	1	150
F		
Figs	1	25
Fig Bar	1	50
Fish, smoked	½	150
Fish Stick	1	50
Fish, sweet & sour	PP	200
Fish, white, broiled	PP	125
fried	PP	225
Flavorings	1 t.	10
Flounder	PP	100
Frankfurter, all beef	1	125
rolls	1	125
French Fried Potatoes	1	15
French Toast	1 sl.	125
Fruit Cocktail	1 c.	100
Fruit Punch	1 gl.	200
Fritters, fruit	1	200
corn	1	100
Fudge	1″ sq.	100

Food	Amount	Pleasure Units
G		
Gefilte fish	1	150
Gelatin-Jello-all flavors	1 c.	100
Ginger Bread	SPP	175
Grapefruit	½	50
Grapes	1 c.	100
Griddle Cakes	PP	100
Gravies, all	1 T.	15
Guavas	1	25
butter	1 T.	50
Guinea Hen	1	175
H		
Haddock	PP	100
Ham	1 sl.	100
deviled	1 T.	100
Hamburger (all beef)	PP	200
fried	PP	225
Hash, corned beef	1 c.	300
Hazel nuts	1	10
Herring	bite size	25
	1 strip	125
creamed	bite size	35
	1 strip	175
Hominy Grits (cooked)	1 c.	75
Honey	1 T.	75
Honeydew Melon	¼	75
Hors d'oeuvres	lg.	50
Horseradish	1 T.	10
Hot Cross Buns	1	150
Hot Dog	1	125
roll	1	125
I		
ICE CREAM		
Ice Cream	1 scoop	150
Ice Milk	1 scoop	100
Fudgsicle	1 bar	100
Popsicle	1 bar	75
Ice Cream Bar	1 bar	200
Cone		175
Sandwich		175
Sundae		400
Banana Split		450
Biscuit Tortoni		175
Cake Roll		175
Indian Nuts	1 T.	25
Italian Bread	½" sl.	50

Food	Amount	Pleasure Units
J		
Jams, Jellies, Preserves, Marma-lade	1 T.	50
Jelly Apple	1	250
Jelly Beans	1	15
Juice, fruit	1 sm. gl.	100
vegetable	1 gl.	75
K		
Kaiser Roll	1	125
Kale	1 c.	50
Kidney Beans	1 c.	225
Kidney/Beef Steak Pie	1 c.	250
Kidney, beef	1 c.	200
lamb	1 c.	125
pie	1 c.	225
Kippered Herring	½	125
Knockwurst	1	200
Kreplach	1	75
Kumquats (fresh)	1	15
L		
Ladyfingers	1	25
Lamb, barbecued	PP	150
chop	1"	250
breast (stewed)	1 c.	200
fried chop	1" thick	325
Lemon	1	25
Lettuce	1 head	50
Lima Beans	1 c.	150
Liver, beef	PP	100
chicken (chopped)	1 scoop	200
paste	1 T.	50
Liverwurst	1 sl.	75
Lobster		
cocktail	1 c.	175
Newburgh	1 c.	150
tail, African	1	100
Loganberries	1 c.	100
London Broil	PP	100
M		
Macaroni (baked)	1 c.	200
with cheese	1 c.	450
Macaroons	1	10
Malted Milk	1 gl.	400
Mango	1	100

Food	Amount	Pleasure Units
Maple Syrup	1 T.	75
Marmalade	1 T.	50
Marshmallow Topping	1 T.	50
Marshmallows	1	25
Matzo	1	75
Matzo Ball	1	125
Mayonnaise	1 T.	100
Meat Balls	1	100
with spaghetti	1 c.	375
Meat Gravy	1 T.	25
Meat Loaf	½" sl.	225
Mexican Rice	1 c.	225
MILK		
Acidophilus	1 gl.	100
Buttermilk	1 gl.	100
Condensed	1 T.	50
Dry-non-fat	1 gl.	75
Evaporated, canned	1 gl.	350
Skim or non-fat	1 gl.	100
Whole	1 gl.	150
Milk Shake	1 gl.	350
Milk Toast	1 sl.	175
Mince pie	TPP	350
Molasses	1 T.	50
Mousse	1 c.	350
Muffins, all	1	150
Mushrooms	1 c.	25
Musscls	10	100
Mustard	1 t.	10
N		
Napoleans	1	300
Navy Beans	1 c.	200
Nectarine	1	50
Noodles, cooked	1 c.	200
Nova Scotia Salmon	1 sl.	200
Nuts, all	sm.	10
	lg.	25
Nuts, Indian	1 T.	25
Litchi	1	10
Pine	1 t.	25
O		
Oils, all	1 T.	125
Orange	1	75
slices	1 c.	100
Omelet	2 eggs, 1 t. but.	185
Onions (boiled)	1	50

Food	Amount	Pleasure Units
creamed	1 c.	150
french fried	1	150
Ovaltine, whole milk	1 c.	225
Oyster cocktail	6	75
fried	1	50
raw	1	10
P		
Pancakes, waffles, & similar break- fast foods	1	150
Pancakes, German	1	225
Parfait	1	225
Parkerhouse Roll	1	100
Party Snacks	sm.	25
	lg.	50
Pastry	each	300
toaster	each	200
Peaches, canned	1	50
fresh	1 med.	50
spiced	1	75
Peanut Brittle	SPP	75
Peanut Butter	1 T.	100
Pear, alligator	1	250
fresh	1 med.	100
Peppers, green (fresh)	1	25
Persian Melons	⅛	75
Persimmons	1 med.	100
Petit Fours	1	100
Pickles, dill or sour	1 sm.	15
or sweet	1 lg.	25
PIES		
Chiffon	TPP	275
Cream	TPP	400
Custard	TPP	200
Fruit	TPP	275
Lemon Meringue	Avg. Piece	350
Pot-Pie, apple	1	500
Pumpkin	TPP	325
Pineapple, crushed	1 c.	150
diced	1 c.	100
sliced	1	25
Pizza	⅙ of 12″ pie, 1 sl.	200
	snack size	25
anchovy	1 sl.	225
sausage	⅛ of 12″ pie, 1 sl.	250
Plum	1	25

Food	Amount	Pleasure Units
Pork Chop	1	225
Pork Fried Rice	1 c.	225
Pork, Kidney	1 c.	150
Pork, liver	PP	150
roast	PP	200
sausage	1	75
sausage patty	1	175
sweet & sour	1 c.	250
Postum (no milk)	1 c.	10
Potato, sweet	1	200
mashed	1 c.	175
hash brown	1 c.	200
Potato Salad	1 c.	350
Potato Pancake	1	175
Potato, lyonnaise	1 c.	400
french fried	1	15
baked	1	125
chips	1	15
sliced, fried	1 c.	500
au gratin	1 c.	400
julienne	1 c.	400
Pot Pies (meat & chicken)	1 whole	400
Pot Roast	PP	150
Pretzel Sticks	1 thin	5
Pretzels	1	20
Prunes (cooked)	1 sm.	25
dried	4	100
Prune Whip	1 c.	100
Puddings	1 c.	400
bread	1 c.	250
rice	1 c.	350
R		
Radishes	1	3
Raspberries	1 c.	100
Rhubarb (stewed—no sugar)	1 c.	50
Rice, brown	1 c.	150
converted, cooked	1 c.	100
chinese, fried	1 c.	200
custard	1 c.	400
fritters	1	50
Roast Beef	PP	100
Rolls	1	100
onion	1	150
plain	1 lg.	150
S		
Salad Dressing	1 T.	75
Salami	¼″ sl.	125

Food	Amount	Pleasure Units
Salmon, baked	PP	250
canned	1 c.	300
loaf	½″ sl.	225
Sauces	1 T.	25
Sauerkraut	1 c.	50
Sausage	1 link	75
Scallops	1	25
Seafood cocktail	1 c.	150
Sherbet, fruit	1 scoop	100
Shish Kebab	1 skewer	350
Shortening	1 T.	100
Shrimp	1	15
fried	1	50
stuffed	1	75
cocktail	6	100
Sirloin Steak	PP	100
tips, beef	PP	100
Smelt (broiled)	1	15
Snapper, Red	PP	100
Sour Cream	1 T.	50
Soda, all soft drinks	1 gl.	100
Sole	PP	100
SOUPS		
Bean	1 c.	150
Bouillon	1 cube	10
Broth (consommé)	1 c.	50
Chicken	1 c.	25
Noodle	1 c.	50
Gumbo	1 c.	100
Rice	1 c.	50
Chowder	1 c.	75
Thick	1 c.	150
Cream Soups	1 c.	150
Pea	1 c.	100
Tomato	1 c.	75
Vegetable	1 c.	75
Vichyssoise	1 c.	100
Soy Beans	1 c.	225
Spaghetti, plain	1 c.	175
with sauce	1 c.	175
with 2 meat balls	1 c.	275
with clam sauce	1 c.	225
Spareribs	1	50
Spinach	1 c.	50
Squash, acorn	1 c.	100
butternut	1 c.	50
summer	1 c.	50

Food	Amount	Pleasure Units
Squid	1 c.	125
Steak, beef	PP	100
Stew, beef	1 c.	250
Strawberries, frozen	1 c.	25
fresh	1	10
Stringbeans	1 c.	25
Strudel, apple	SPP	225
Sturgeon	PP	150
Sugar	1 t.	20
Sukiyaki	1 c.	250
Sweet Potato	1	200
Sweet Potato Pie	TPP	450
Sweet Rolls	1	125
Sweetbreads	1 c.	250
Syrups	1 T.	75
T		
Tangerines	1	50
Tomato (fresh)	1 med.	25
juice	1 c.	50
aspic	1 c.	50
Tongue, beef	PP of 1 sl.	50
TOPPINGS		
Butterscotch	1 T.	50
Caramel	1 T.	50
Chocolate	1 T.	75
Pineapple	1 T.	50
Fudge	1 T.	75
Whipped Cream	1 T.	10
Trout	PP	100
Tuna Fish (in oil)	1 c.	400
water packed	1 c.	250
Turkey	PP	125
Turnovers, apple	1	250
V		
Veal Cutlets	PP	100
breaded	PP	150
with cheese & tomato (Parm.)	PP	350
chop	½″ thick	150
Marsala	PP	200
Scalloppine	PP	250
stew	1 c.	250
Vinegar	1 oz.	0
VEGETABLES		
Asparagus	1 c.	25
Lima Beans	1 c.	200

Food	Amount	Pleasure Units
Broccoli	1 c.	50
Brussels Sprouts	1 c.	50
Cabbage	1 c.	25
Cauliflower	1 c.	25
Carrots	1 c.	50
Eggplant	1 c.	50
Peas	1 c.	100
Potatoes	1 c.	175
Spinach	1 c.	50
Squash	1 c.	100
W		
Waffle	1	225
Water		0
Watermelon	TPP	50
balls	1 c.	50
Wax Beans	1 c.	25
Whipped Cream	1 T.	50
Whitefish, smoked	½	150
Wiener schnitzel	PP	300
Won Ton	1	100
Worcestershire Sauce	1 T.	25
Yams	1	200
Yogurt, plain	1 c.	175
Z		
Zabaglione	1 c.	150
Zweiback	1	35

The Pleasure Unit List is presented in alphabetical order. In order to make it easy to use, many items in a particular category have been grouped together. For example, *"Alcoholic Beverages"* contain all representative drinks such as beer, wine, cocktails, etc. *"Beverages, Common,"* list almost all drinks such as soda, milk, malts, etc. Cakes, Candy, Cookies, Crackers, Ice Cream, Pies, Soups and Toppings have all been listed in a similar manner as general categories. Though a specific food may not be listed under a category, a typical example should be found. If you wish to find a ham sandwich, look up ham, bread, lettuce and mayonnaise and add them up. Various kinds of potatoes will be listed under "Potato," i.e., Potato, lyonnaise. Read through the list so you can become familiar with it and, therefore, quickly find the foods you want. If a particular dish is not listed, estimate the individual ingredients and add them up.

ABBREVIATIONS AND DEFINITIONS

1 t.	=	1 teaspoon	= ⅙ oz.
1 T.	=	1 tablespoon	= ½ oz.
1 c.	=	1 tea cup	= 6 oz.
1 sm. gl.	=	1 juice glass	= 4 oz.
1 gl.	=	1 glass	= 8 oz.
1 sl.	=	1 slice (standard)	= Packaged cheese, bread, salami, ham, etc.
1 PP	=	1 Pleasure Portion	= Portion the size of the palm of your hand; ¼" thick.
1 TPP	=	Triangular Pleasure Portion	= Measured by creating an imaginary triangle between the thumb and index finger.
1 SPP	=	Square Pleasure Portion	= Measured by forming a right angle between the thumb and index finger. Base is the thumb length. Side is to the first joint of index finger.

Remember: If you fry, add 50.
If you bread, add 50.

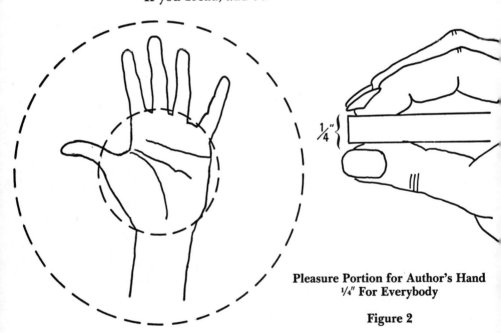

Pleasure Portion for Author's Hand
¼" For Everybody

Figure 2

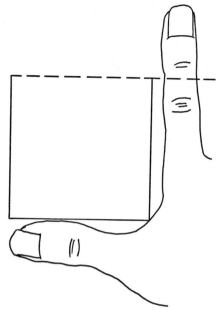

Figure 3—SPP

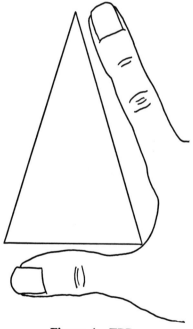

Figure 4—TPP

Pleasure Portion (abbreviated PP). A piece of food, one-quarter-inch thick (which you can estimate), the size of the palm of your hand. The palm of your hand should be represented by an imaginary circle the diameter of which extends from the base of your fingers to the beginning of your wrist.

A Square Pleasure Portion. Measured by holding thumb and index finger at right angles. The base is equal to the length of your thumb and the sides to level of the knuckle of the index finger. Used for measuring cakes and puddings.

A Triangular (wedge-shape) Pleasure Portion. Measured by creating an imaginary triangle between the thumb and index finger. Used for measuring pies and cakes.

EXCHANGE LISTS (PLEASURE UNIT PLANS)

Some people just hate to have total control over their lives and must be given a game plan to simplify matters. For those who want guidance, I offer two choices:

Ultra Simple

1. Count your pleasure units.
2. Eat a lot of vegetables.
3. Eat meat only once a day.
4. Eat fish or chicken more often.
5. Hold down the simple sugars, flour products, and fats.

Simple

Use the exchange lists supplied to lose or maintain weight. They will guide you to a balanced nourishing diet.

1000 PLEASURE UNIT PLAN

Food	Number of Pleasure Portions	Exchange List
Milk	2	1a
Vegetables	2–4	2a
Fruits	2	3
Bread	4	4

Protein Foods
   Animal   4   5a
   Vegetable   1   2c,d, 5a
Fats   3   6
Free Foods   As Desired (AD)   7

Typical Meal Pattern

Breakfast

1 Milk 1a
1 Fruit 3
1 Bread 4a
1 Fat 6

Lunch

1 Milk (A1) 1a
At least 1 vegetable (B) 2a
1 Fruit (D) 3
2 Bread (E) 4
2 Animal Protein (F1) 5a
1 Vegetable Protein (G1,2) (or at lunch) 2c,d
1 Fat (H) 6

Dinner

At least 1 Vegetable (B) 2a
1 Bread (E) 4
2 Animal Protein (F1) 5a
1 Vegetable Protein (G1,2) (or at lunch) 2c,d
1 Fat (H) 6
Snack

AD Free Foods (I) 7

2000 PLEASURE UNIT PLAN

Food	*Number of Pleasure Portions*	*Exchange List*
Milk	2	1b
Vegetables		
Low-calorie	2–4	2a

2000 PLEASURE UNIT PLAN (Cont.)

Moderate calorie	2	2b
Fruits	6	3
Bread	9	4
Protein Foods		
Animal	5	5a
Vegetable	1	2c,d–
		5a
Fats	8	6
Free Foods	As Desired (AD)	7

Typical Meal Pattern

Breakfast

1 Serving Milk 1b
2 Servings Fruit 3
3 Servings Bread 4
2 Servings Fat 6

Lunch

1 Serving Milk (A2) 1b
At least 1 Serving Vegetable (B) 2a
2 Servings Fruit (D) 3
2 Servings Bread (E) 4
2 Servings Animal Protein (F1) 5a
1 Serving Vegetable Protein (G1,2) (or at dinner) 2c,d, 5a
3 Servings Fat (H) 6

Dinner

At least 1 Serving Vegetable (B) 2a
2 Servings Vegetable (C) 2b
2 Servings Bread (E) 4
3 Servings Animal Protein (F1) 5a
1 Serving Vegetable Protein (G1,2) (or at lunch) 2c,d, 5a

Snack

2 Servings Fruit (D) 3
2 Servings Bread (E) 4
AD Free Foods (I) 7

EXCHANGE LISTS

LIST 1a   *Milk Exchange*   *100 Pleasure Units*

	Amount
Non-Fat	1 gl.
Skim milk	
Powdered (non-fat, dry) milk	⅓ c.
Buttermilk made from skim milk	1 gl.
Canned, evaporated, skim milk	½ c.
Yogurt made from skim milk (plain)	1 c.

LIST 1b   *125 Pleasure Units*

Low-Fat

Low-fat milk (2% fat)	1 gl.
Yogurt made from low-fat milk	1 c.

LIST 1c   *150 Pleasure Units*

Whole milk	1 gl.
Canned, evaporated, whole milk	1 gl.
Powdered milk	1 gl.
Buttermilk made from whole milk	1 c.
Yogurt made from whole milk (plain)	1 c.

LIST 2a   *Vegetable Exchange–25 Pleasure Units*

Low Pleasure Units—1 c. Raw—½ c. cooked

Asparagus	Greens:	Rhubarb
Bamboo shoots	Beets	(unsweetened)
Bean sprouts	Chards	Sauerkraut
Beans, green or wax	Collards	Scallions
Broccoli	Dandelion	Squash (summer)
Brussels sprouts	Kale	Casserta
Cabbage	Mustard	Chayote
Cauliflower	Spinach	Cymling
Celery	Turnip	Pattypan
Chicory	Jicama root	Scalloped
Chinese cabbage	Lettuce	Spaghetti
Chives	Mushrooms	Straight or Crook-neck
Cucumbers	Okra	Zucchini
Eggplant	Onion	Tomatoes (limited to
Endive	Parsley	½ c. or 1 medium
Escarole	Pea pods	Watercress
Fennel	Peppers, green or red	Wintermelon
	Radishes	

LIST 2b   *Vegetable Exchange*   *50 Pleasure Units*

High Pleasure Units—1c. Raw—½ c. cooked

Artichoke	Pumpkin	Danish
Beets	Rutabaga	Des Moines
Carrots	Squash (winter)	Hubbard
Kohlrabi	Acorn	Tomato juice
Onions	Banana	Tomato paste
Parsnips	Butternut	(¼ cup)
		Turnips

LIST 2c   *Vegetable Products*   *Low-Fat—150 Pleasure Units*

Amount

Dried beans, peas (cooked, drained)
includes kidney, lima, navy, pinto,
split peas, black-eyed peas, lentils,
garbanzo, red, pink, black, broad,
cow peas, mung, white   ¾ c.
Soups   ¾ c.

LIST 2d   *100 Pleasure Units*

Medium Fat

Soybeans (cooked)   ½ c.
Tofu   ⅔ c.

LIST 2e   *200 Pleasure Units*

High Fat

Nuts, seeds   2 T.
Peanut butter   2 T.

LIST 3   *Fruit Exchange*   *100 Pleasure Units*

Amount

Fruits   2 pcs.
small, all dried   4 pcs.
Juice, fruit   1 sm. gl.
vegetable   1 gl.

LIST 3—*Fruit Exchange (Cont.)*

	Amount
Berries, all kinds	1 c.
Cherries	20
Melons, Cantaloupe	½" wedge
Honeydew	¼" wedge
Watermelon	2" wedge
Raisins	4 T.

LIST 4a *Bread Exchange* *100 Pleasure Units*

	Amount
Bread	1 sl.
French	1 sl.
Pumpernickel	1 sl.
Rye	1 sl.
White	1 sl.
Whole Wheat	1 sl.
Bread cubes, dry	½ c.
Bread crumbs, dry	3 T.
Biscuit (omit 1 fat exchange)	1
Boston brown	1 sl.
Bagel	½
Cornbread (omit 1 fat exchange)	1 ½ in. cube
Corn muffin (omit 1 fat exchange)	1 (2-in. diameter)
Hamburger bun	½
Hot dog bun	½
Muffin (omit 1 fat exchange)	1
Muffin, English	½
Pita Bread	¼ (7-in. diameter)
Roll, dinner	1 (2-in. diameter)
Taco Shell	1
Tortilla, flour, corn	1 (6-in. diameter)
Cereals	
Bran flakes	½ c.
Cereal, cooked	½ c.
Cereal, puffed (unfrosted)	1 c.
Cereal, ready-to-eat, unsweetened	¾ c.
Cornmeal, dry	2 T
Granola (omit 1 fat exchange)	¼ c.
Crackers	
Arrowroot	3
Graham	2 (2½ in. sq.)
Matzo	½
Oyster	20 (⅓ c.)
Melba toast	1 sl.
Pretzels	20
Rounds, thin	6

LIST 4a—Bread Exchange (Cont.)

	Amount
Rye wafers	3
Saltines	6
Soda	4
Barley, cooked	½ c.
Corn	⅓ c.
Crepe	1 (6-in. diameter)
Pancake	1
Pasta (cooked)	
Noodles	½ c.
Macaroni	½ c.
Spaghetti	½ c.
Potato	
French Fries (omit 1 fat exchange)	8
Sweet or Yams	¼ c.
White (baked, boiled)	1 sm.
White (mashed)	½ c.
Popcorn (no butter)	3 cups
Rice (cooked)	½ c.
Waffle	1
Wheat bran	4 T.
Wheat germ	4 T.
Goodies	
Cake, angel food, sponge (no icing), coffee, or crumb, cupcake	1 SPP
Cookies	
Arrowroot	4
Fig bar	1
Gingersnap	2
Vanilla wafers	3
Cornstarch	2 T.
Flour	2½ T.
Marshmallows	4
Potato or corn chips (omit 2 fat exchanges)	15
Mints	10
Chocolate covered mints	3
Lollipop	1
Chocolate kisses	4
Jelly Beans	10
Bon Bons	2
Candied fruit	1
Caramels	2
Gum Drops	6
Life Savers	8

LIST 4a—Bread Exchange (Cont.)

	Amount
Sugar, syrups	5 t.
Tapioca	2 T.

LIST 4b   Extra Goodies   300 Pleasure Units

Cakes
    Cheese   TPP
    Chocolate   TPP
    Coconut   TPP
    Devil's Food   ½" sl.
    Eclair   1
    Honey   1" sl.
    Jelly Roll   ¾" sl.
    Marble   1" sl.
    Pound   1" sl.
    Sponge   1" sl.
    Strawberry Shortcake   TPP
    Strudel   1
    Upside Down   SPP
    Whipped Cream   TPP
    All other cakes with icing   TPP
Candy
    All chocolate or chocolate
    covered candy bars   1

List 5a   Protein Exchange   100 Pleasure units   Pleasure Portion

Lean Meat

Beef:	Baby beef, chipped beef, chuck flank steak, tenderloin, plate ribs, plate skirt steak, round, rump, sirloin, tripe, shank
Lamb:	Leg, rib, sirloin, loin (roast and chops), shank, shoulder
Pork:	Leg (whole rump, center shank); ham, smoked
Veal:	Leg, loin, rib, shank, shoulder, cutlets
Poultry:	Meat without skin of chicken, turkey, cornish hen, guinea hen, pheasant, rabbit
Seafood:	Cod, flounder, haddock, halibut, perch, sea bass, sole, tuna canned in water, abalone, crayfish, octopus, scallops, shrimp, squid, turtle, catfish, smelts, sturgeon, fresh tuna, clams, crab, lobster, mussels, oysters, scrod

Cheeses containing less than 5% butterfat
Cottage cheese, dry curd and 2% butterfat

LIST 5b   *150 Pleasure Units*   *Pleasure Portion*

Medium Fat

Beef:	Ground (15% fat) corned beef
Pork:	Loin (all cuts), tenderloin, shoulder arm, shoulder blade (Boston butt), canadian bacon, boiled ham, picnic ham, pigs feet Liver, heart, kidney, and sweetbreads (these are high in cholesterol—eggs)
Fish:	Albacore, carp, salmon, tuna (canned in oil, drained)
Cheese:	Cottage cheese, creamed, Ricotta (part skim), Mozzarella (part skim), Neufchatel, farmer cheese

LIST 5c   *200 Pleasure Units*   *Pleasure Portion*

High Fat

Beef:	Corned beef (brisket), ground beef (more than 20% fat), chuck, (ground commercial), roasts (rib), steaks (club and rib), Pastrami
Lamb:	Breast
Pork:	Spare ribs, loin (back ribs), ground, country-style ham, deviled ham, bacon, salt pork
Veal:	Breast
Poultry:	Capon, duck (domestic), goose
Fish:	Anchovies, herring, mackerel, sardines, shad, trout, tuna (canned in oil), eel
Cheese:	Whole milk Ricotta, Cheddar, Cream, Gruyève, Brick, Jack, Swiss, American, Blue, Feta, Parmesan, Romano, Brie, Colby, Gjetost, Muenster, Portsalut, Roquefort, Cheshire, processed cheese spread, Provolone, Gouda, Limburger, Edam, Camembert, Tilsit, whole milk Mozzarella
Cold cuts	1 sl.
Frankfurter	1
Sausage	1
Salami	1

LIST 6   *50 Pleasure Units*

Fat Exchange	*Amount*
Polyunsaturated Fat:	
Mayonnaise	1 t.
Oil	1 t.
Corn	
Cottonseed	
Safflower	
Soybean	
Sunflower	

LIST 6   *Fat Exchange (Cont.)*

Fat Exchange	*Amount*
Wheat germ	
Salad Dressing	
Clear type (oil & vinegar), regular	1 T.
Clear type (oil & vinegar), low-cal.	3 T.
Mayonnaise type, regular	1 T.
Mayonnaise type, low-cal.	2 T.
Soft margarine	1 t.
Soybean lecithin	1 t.

Monounsaturated Fat

Avocado	⅛ (4 in. diameter)
Guacamole dip	2 T.
Non-dairy creamer, liquid	2 T.
Nuts, all	5 small
	3 large
Nut butters	1 t.
Nut, chopped	1 T.
Olives	5 small
Olive oil	1 t.
Peanut oil	1 t.
Seeds	1 T.
Pumpkin	
Sesame	
Sunflower	
Seed butters	1 t.
Shortening	1 t.
Stick margarine	1 t.

Saturated Fat

Bacon fat	1 t.
Butter	1 t.
Cocoa butter	1 t.
Coconut oil	1 t.
Coconut, shredded, unsweetened	1 T.
Cream cheese	1 T.
Cream	
Half-and-Half	3 T.
Light, sour	2 T.
Whipped, unsweetened	2 T.
Whipping, heavy	1 T.
Lard	1 t.
Non-dairy creamer, powdered	5 t.

List 7   Free Foods   No Pleasure Units

Beverages

Bouillon (without fat)
Carbonated beverages unsweetened or artificially sweetened
Coffee
Consommé (without fat)
Diet drinks
Mineral waters
Tea

Food

Celery
Chicory
Chinese cabbage
Cucumbers
Endive

Escarole
Gelatin, unsweetened
    or artificially sweetened
Lettuce
Pickles, unsweetened
Watercress

Seasonings (No Salt)

Allspice
Almond extract
Anise seed
Basil
Bay leaf
Bouillon cube,
    low-sodium dietetic
Caraway seed
Cardamon
Cassia
Celery; leaves or seed
Chervil
Chili powder (no added
    salt)
Chives
Cilantro
Cinnamon
Cloves
Coriander
Cumin
Curry
Garlic; juice or powder
Ginger

Horseradish root, or pre-
    pared without salt
Juniper
Lemon juice or extract
Lime
Mace
Maple extract
Marjoram
Meat tenderizers; low-
    sodium dietetic
Mint
Mustard, dry or seed
Nutmeg
Onion, juice, powder
Orange extract
Oregano
Paprika
Parsley, leaf or flakes
Pepper, fresh; green or red
Pepper black, red, or white
Peppermint extract
Pimento peppers
Poppyseed

Poultry season-
    ing (no salt
    added)
Pumpkin spice
Purslane
Rosemary
Saffron
Sage
Salt substitutes (if
    recommended
    by your physi-
    cian)
Savory
Sorrel
Tarragon
Thyme
Turmeric
Vanilla extract
Vinegar
Walnut extract
Wine, table, (in
    cooking)

Seasonings (High Salt)

Baking powder, soda
Bouillon cube, regular
Celery salt
Chili sauce
Garlic salt
Horseradish; uncreamed,
  prepared with salt
Meat extracts
Meat tenderizers
Monosodium glutamate

Mustard; prepared
Onion salt
Pickles; unsweetened
Salt
Seasoning salts
Soy sauce
Tabasco sauce
Wine (in cooking)
Worcestershire sauce

LIST 8   *Miscellaneous*   *100 Pleasure Units*

Beverages	*Amount*
Ale, beer, malt	1 gl.
Cocktail	2½ oz.
Highball	¾ gl.
Whiskey	1½ oz.
Wine & Champagne	3 oz.
Eggnog	3 oz.
Milk	¾ gl.
Chocolate milk	½ gl.
Shakes	¾ oz (a whole glass would be 500 Pleasure Units— so think twice or even 3 times

Scene 3
Pleasure Begets Pleasure

I know a physician in his late thirties who gets up every morning at five o'clock, tapes his ankles, puts on a sweat suit and special sneakers, and then runs twelve miles. He told me it takes about an hour and a half. After running, he goes to the the hospital on rounds and then to the office to see his patients. As we talked, I must admit I had mixed feelings about him. While I openly admired (and was secretly jealous of) his physical ability, I felt he must be weird to do that every day. I could never see myself doing that; I'd be bored to tears.

When the exercise craze first began, I had to drive extra carefully both to and from work. Everywhere I went, I saw people jogging, walking, and riding bicycles. Nowadays, however, I rarely see anyone exercising except for a small group of dedicated athletes, including one eighty-year-old man who walks rapidly every morning, with spindly legs protruding from his gym shorts and wearing an expression which seems to tell me he is trying to reach the watering hole before he drops dead. Aside from these people who enjoy (?) their workouts, and those afraid of the possible consequences of not exercising, the physical fitness "fad" seems to have run its course.

While exercising is no longer extremely popular, keeping the body in shape is still extremely important and there is no question that a program of activity is beneficial. There are two big problems however. First, unless people like what they are doing, the odds are probably a hundred to one that they will not continue doing it. The second problem is that while you may enjoy playing sports like football in your teens and early twenties, they become too dangerous and difficult when you become older. A fair number of individuals may truly enjoy tennis, and be able to play it for thirty or forty years, but the majority will stop long before that and only the rare exception will continue longer. Yet the

176

need for body activity and recreation continues throughout life. Walking and swimming seem to have the longest life span of any activity, and you can add bicycle ridng if you consider that you can start with a tricycle and end up with a tricycle. These are three generally beneficial activities and probably the best. In recent years, medical authorities with support of the government and industry, worked very hard to encourage greater activity in our progressively sedentary society. Though great strides have been made, I would suspect the overall result disappointing. As I see it, the overall results are similar to those achieved in weight-reduction; the public loses weight, the public becomes more active. After a short period of time, the public becomes sedentary, and the public regains the weight. It is for this reason that I feel the Pleasure Principle will provide an answer for millons of individuals.

PLEASURE UNIT CREDITS

Consider for a moment the average amount of activity that you do each day. Everything you do burns up energy. If you slept twenty-four hours a day, you would burn up approximately a 1000 to 1500 Pleasure Units. Anything you do above and beyond sleeping will burn up more energy. How can this fact be used to an advantage in the "Pleasure Principle?" The first sentence in the *Pleasure Principle* is "seek only pleasure." Now if anything that you do is more active than sleeping, and will burn up more energy, then anything pleasurable you do, other than sleeping, will burn up even more energy. Before there is a misunderstanding, I do advocate a good night's sleep. However, it's with your waking hours that I offer you double the pleasure. Before I go any further, I am going to ask you to do something and I want you to take it seriously. I would like you to put this book down, take a pencil and a piece of paper, and list all of the things that you like to do. I'm not just talking about sports or gymnastics or walking, I'm talking about anything that you like to do including reading, playing cards, dancing, painting, sewing your own clothes, volunteering at your local hospital or debating society, and so on. Oh yes, and don't forget sex. After you have made your list, I have a surprise for you on the next page.

Start listing!

Did you peek?

If so, you've got one more chance to be honest.

Now that you've made your list, you can turn to the surprise on the next page.

If you will do any of the activities that you have listed, more *than you usually do them, your pleasure will beget pleasure. In other words, the more pleasure you have, the more pleasure you will get, or as they say, double your pleasure, double your fun.*

Let me explain further. You are living at a certain average pace at the present time, burning up so much energy every day. *If you will start doing the things that give you pleasure more than you have done them before, you will increase your pleasure in life three ways.*

1. You will have *more pleasure*, because you are doing more of the things that you like to do.
2. You will have *more pleasure*, because you are burning up more energy and *losing weight faster*.
3. You could lose weight at the same rate, and have *more pleasure* by taking the Pleasure Units that you gain as credits from doing more activity, and *spend it on food that gives you pleasure*.

I have listed below many everyday activities and the number of Pleasure Unit Credits you can earn for every fifteen minutes that you spend doing these activities. If I have omitted anything that you have listed, find something on my list that closely approximates the kind of activity you like to do and use the same number of units.

It is not necessary for any activity to be strenuous in order for you to gain Pleasure Credits and control your weight more efficiently. In fact, moderate activity is advised. The increase in your activity should be on a daily basis. After all, why should you only have fun on weekends. It is also advisable to vary the kind of activity that you do, otherwise you are liable to turn something very pleasurable into a boring chore. Activities which are continuous, rather than stop-and-go, are far more beneficial. Because walking is such a natural everyday thing (at least it used to be), it would be a great idea to get used to walking as much as possible. Try to do it in ways that are pleasant and fun. It will break up the monotony of each day. For example, if you drive to work and park in the company parking lot, you could avoid the frustrating jam-up at the end of the day by parking several blocks away and walking. If that isn't feasible, you might jog to your car in the parking lot and burn up a little more energy that way.

If you like to do calisthenics, fine; I've included a description of a few of them that you might enjoy doing that will tone up your muscles. If, however, you don't enjoy calisthenics, I have also included a description of some simple isometrics that you can do anywhere, anytime, and nobody will even know that you are doing them. They not only burn up extra energy, but they will help you in tightening up your thighs, tummy, and chest muscles.

Most mechanical devices are a waste of time and money. The chances are you will use them for only a few weeks and they will just stand there taking up space in your closet. I'm sure the money could be spent on something more pleasurable. Stay away from the gimmick devices such as rubber suits, electrical belts, and the like. They have been proven to be worthless and could even be harmful.

An activity program is not something you are going to be involved in just while you are losing weight. Make it a part of the "Pleasure Principle" so that it becomes a way of living. Remember, that as you get older there is a tendency to slow down and gaining weight back becomes easier. If you learn to increase your activity in a thousand little *pleasurable* ways, this is less likely to happen.

There are some unusual ways in which you can increase your pleasure and activity, and lessen some of the boring or upsetting moments in your life. For example, if you are watching television and a commercial that you've seen a hundred times interrupts your favorite program, why don't you get up and dance to the jingle? If there is no music, you could increase your activity by getting up and walking out of the room; it might be even more fun to stand in front of the television set, making faces and poking fun at whomever is taking part in the commercial.

Are you one of those people who cannot seem to relax? If you increase your activity and enjoy yourself more, you will find that you will be able to relax better. After all, whenever you stop the extra activity, you will be relaxing. Don't equate work with pleasurable activity (unless you enjoy your work that much). Usually work is accomplished under some stress and strain, physically and mentally. Pleasurable activity though, is accomplished with a good frame of mind and with your muscles far less tense. It will increase your circulation and invigorate you. You know how good it feels to stretch when you get up in the morning or if you have been sitting for long hours at a time. Why not make it a practice to frequently move your arms and legs and wiggle your fingers and toes. I had the pleasure of meeting a bright young woman who is writing a doctoral thesis in physical education at Walden University. She described a technique of getting severely handicapped patients in nursing homes to take part in group activities. She would play all kinds of music tapes for them, and have them move any part of their body that they could in rhythm to the music. She told me that some of the patients were so severely handicapped that all they could do was blink their eyes or smile in rhythm to the music. You could try this while driving in your car. If you listen to one of those all-news programs, you could even move in rhythm to their talking; don't worry what the other drivers will think.

The beneficial process of developing better posture will also burn up more energy. The easiest way I know of is to "think tall" whether you are sitting, standing, or walking. Think tall. You will find that your head comes up, your chest automatically comes out, your belly goes in, and you look better. In addition, you may be preventing some serious problems with your spine and circulation.

When you learn to think tall, your spine will straighten and your posture will improve markedly. Stand in front of the mirror and do this and you will see what I mean. Don't assume the military posture, that's exaggerated and awkward, and is not something that you can do for any length of time. But thinking tall and raising your head high is something that you can remind yourself of all day long. Another technique for improving your physical appearance is to learn to pull your stomach in, especially while talking if at all possible, that's the hardest way. At first you might think in terms of using reminders. When the telephone rings, or stopped at a red light, or while brushing your teeth . . . pull in your stomach. If you start doing this, you will find that your abdominal muscles become much firmer. You'll start saving money and girdles.

Remember, you can only count as Pleasure Credits the activity you will be doing that is in excess of the activity you normally do. With these extra Pleasure Credits you can either have extra delicious bites of dessert or whatever it is that you like, or you can save the credits and lose weight faster.

Let's talk about one of my favorite subjects, sex. If you are having sexual relations twice a week now, and you have sexual relations four times a week from now on, you can accumulate 500 Pleasure Credits each week, which you can spend or save. That's 250 credits . . . pleasure begets pleasure! I am sure some reader is going to come up with the unique approach of calling a friend on the phone and saying, "Hi there, I'm trying to lose weight, do you want to help me get some extra Pleasure Credits?" It may sound strange, but with all of the emphasis that the U.S. Department of Health and Human Services has been placing on increased physical activity, why haven't they encouraged more sexual activity? Now for some of you who have heard bad rumors about the effect of sex on the heart, and possibly have heard about someone who "died with their boots on," let me present an interesting fact. A number of years ago I read a medical article involving research done with avionics. Avionics is a technique in which a small electrocardiogram is strapped to the chest and a twenty-four hour recording of heart activity is made. The subjects of this research were asked to mark down on a sheet, all of the activities and incidents that occurred during a twenty-four hour period, and the times at which they occurred. The subjects included eating meals, running for buses, work, exercise, reading telegrams, etc. What do you think had the most serious effect on the heart as indicated by changes on the cardiogram? Answer: Having an argument at the dinner table with your children. What do you think was included among the least affecting activities on the cardiogram? Answer: Sexual intercourse!!

For those of you who have had heart attacks, a frank discussion with your family doctor or cardiologist is strongly suggested. There is a reason for this. Sexual activity, in itself, is not contraindicated, but certain types of sexual activity might be best avoided. One of the frequently suggested changes in technique of enjoying sex may be somewhat demoralizing to the male chauvinist. If the man has had a heart attack, it is often preferable for the woman to "get on top" during sex play. Don't be narrow minded; "Try it, you might like it!"

The Pleasure Principle can also be helpful in breaking some bad habits. Very often when people try to give up smoking, they trade one treacherous habit for another, overeating. It's not giving up smoking that causes the excess weight to accumulate, it's merely the substitution of eating for smoking. Why not try gaining some extra Pleasure Unit Credits by substituting one of your fun activities for smoking. A better title for the list that you made would be the "Fun and Diversion List." However, if you are giving up smoking and you decide to eat instead, remember to take out your pad and pencil and write it down, before you eat it.

PLEASURE CREDIT ACTIVITY LIST
(Fun and Diversion List)

This list is provided to add fun to your life, increase your physical health and improve your emotional well-being. With it, you can earn Pleasure Credits and divert your attention when the inappropriate unhealthy urge to overeat comes upon you. By all means eat, only when you have the units to spend. However, if you're running out of units, you might enjoy life more by doing the following:

Get involved in club activities.
Call a friend.
Write a book (but not on diets—please).
Play with the kids in a schoolyard or park.
Walk the dog, carry the cat, or just walk.
Watch television.
Build models.
Volunteer at a hospital or nursing home.
Shower with a friend (see below).

I have tried to group activities into categories such as sports, hobbies, daily living, housework, etc. I had difficulty classifying sex, as it could fall under any and all classifications, depending upon the individual. As a sex educator, I have taken the privilege of putting sex first, in a class all by itself, where I think it rightly belongs.

Remember, these activities must be in addition to your usual routine!

Pleasure Activity	Pleasure Credits (For time spent)		Comments
	15 min.	1 hour	
Sexual intercourse and sex play	125	500	Suggested minimum ½ hour or 250 credits
Resting (bed)	15	60	
Sitting	20	80	
Dressing	25	100	
Eating	25	100	
Kneeling	25	100	
Standing	25	100	
Driving a car	25	100	It's twice as good to walk
Showering	50	200	It pays to keep clean
General light activity	50	200	
Walking (indoors)	50	200	
Walking (outdoors)	75	300	
Walking (downstairs)	100	400	Try the Empire State building
Walking (upstairs)	300	1200	
Earning a Living			
Office work (active)	35	140	Whistle while you work
Manual labor (light)	75	300	
Manual labor (heavy)	150	600	
Housework (turn it into housepleasure)			
Sweeping	25	100	
Doing the laundry	50	200	
Making beds	50	200	
Cooking	50	200	
Mopping floors	75	300	
Scrubbing floors	100	400	
Home Repairs			
Woodwork, brickwork, gardening	100	400	
Hobbies			
Painting	25	100	
Playing cards	25	100	
Piano playing	25	100	
Writing	25	100	

Pleasure Activity	Pleasure Credits (For time spent)		Comments
	15 min.	*1 hour*	
Knitting	25	100	
Typing	25	100	
Crocheting	25	100	
Sewing	25	100	
Making model airplanes, boats, etc.	25	100	
Ceramics			
Light gardening	50	200	
Carpentry	75	300	
Sports			
Running	300	1200	If you don't enjoy it, get a gorilla to chase you.
Jogging	200	800	Join a friend, he may be lonesome
Skiing	200	800	
Football	150	600	Make it boys against girls, who knows, there may be an extra 250 credits in it for you.
Baseball	100	400	
Basketball	100	400	
Bicycling	100	400	When going uphill, double the credits
Rowing	100	400	
Tennis	100	400	
Walking briskly	100	400	
Golf	75	300	No golf carts allowed
Bowling	75	300	
Ping-Pong	75	300	
Skating	75	300	
Fast Dancing	75	300	
Volleyball	75	300	
Walking	50	200	
Billiards	50	200	
Badminton	50	200	
Sailing	50	200	Add an extra 50, if you run aground and get free by yourself.
Horseback Riding	50	200	Multiply by 50, if you let the horse get on top
Slow Dancing	50	200	A great opportunity to go for an extra 500 credits

If you have some activity that is not listed, pick one that is similar from those above and use those credits listed.

All activities should be done at an average pace without overexertion.

OCEANS OF MOTIONS

The following is a description of body movements which will burn up energy, increase circulation and limber up your joints and muscles. They can be done at various times during the day and not take away time from anything else you like to do. Some can be done while lying in bed; others can be accomplished while watching television, driving your car, waiting for a bus, talking on the telephone, or preparing meals. Choose the appropriate motion for the proper moment, otherwise some people will think you ought to be put away somewhere even though there is no law against any of them. Don't worry about them, though; it's their problem, not yours!

Motions

There are always moments during the day when the following movements can be done inconspicuously. If they come to take you away, you can always break down and tell them the truth. If they don't believe you, tell them to call me; however, I will not accept collect calls.

Number/minute = pleasure credits earned per minute.

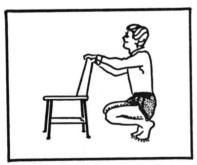

Do knee bends, using a chair if you'd like (50/minute).

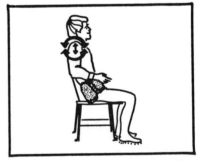

While sitting or standing, shrug your shoulders up and down, backwards and forward, and round and round (20/minute).

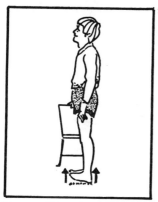

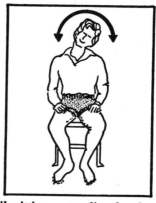

While standing, lift up your toes and feet putting your weight on your heels; then come down and stand up on your toes (20/minute).

While sitting or standing, bend your head forward, backward, side to side, and roll it around in circles (20/minute).

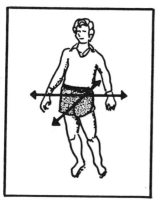

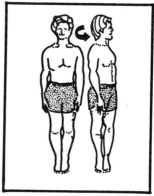

Twist your pelvis from side to side, backward and forward. This is great with music! (30/minute).

Instead of turning your head from side to side, twist your body at the waist (30/minute).

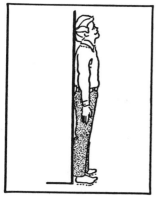

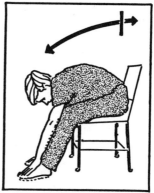

Instead of leaning against a wall, try and get your entire back flat against it and take deep breaths (2/minute).

While sitting or standing, bend over and touch your toes. Straighten up and repeat (3/minute).

Earn Pleasure Credits at home, at work, or even while waiting for a bus.

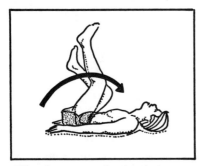

Bicycle on your back (4/minute).

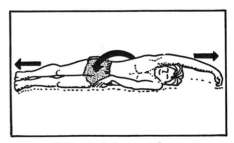

Stretch your right arm above your head and stretch your right leg straight out as far as possible. Roll to your left side and back again. Repeat with the left arm and leg (2/ minute).

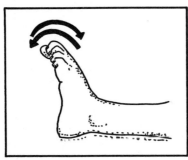

While sitting or lying down, curl your toes and then stretch them back (2/minute).

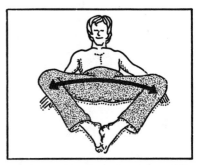

Let your knees fall apart while keeping the soles of your feet facing each other and touching (2/ minute).

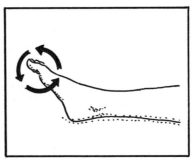

Rotate your foot in circles (2/minute).

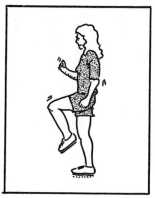

Jog or run in place every chance you get (10/minute).

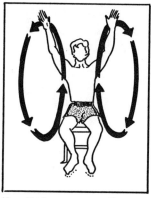

While siitting or standing, rotate your outstretched arms in big circles (3/minute).

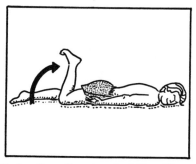

Lying face down and while taking deep breaths, alternately bend both knees and touch your buttocks (2/minute).

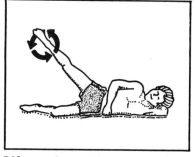

Lift one leg while lying on your side and make circles in the air. Repeat with the other leg (3/minute).

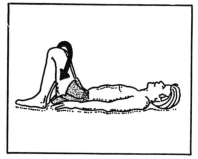

Bend your knees up and let them fall from side to side (3/minute).

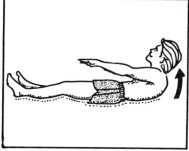

Lie on your back and stretch both arms above your head. Take in a deep breath, and as you exhale, bring your arms forward toward your toes. If you can sit up and touch your toes, so much the better (5/minute).

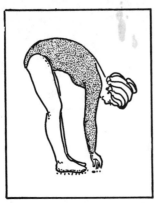

Drop ten pennies and pick them up one at a time (5/minute).

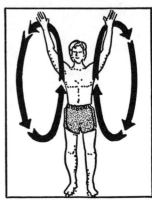

When you can see the bus in the distance, wave it down with both arms (3/minute).

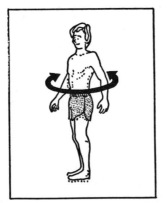

Turn from side to side, looking over your shoulder, to see if the bus is coming (3/minute).

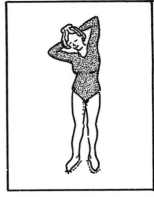

You might pretend you're stretching because the bus is taking so long to arrive (some people won't have to pretend) (3/minute).

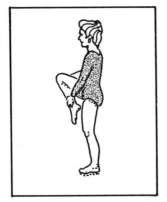

Bend up your knee as though you were rubbing a sore ankle. Check the other ankle while you're at it (3/minute).

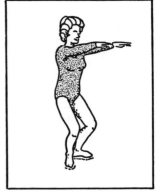

This is a half knee-bend, you might pretend you're scratching your leg (scratch for 10 seconds) (4/minute).

These are great when you're in bed or on the floor watching television. They can be done in the park, at the beach, or in your backyard.

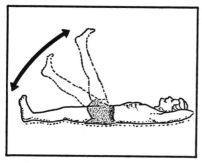

Raise legs alternately and lower them slowly (4/minute).

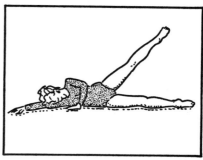

Lie on your right side and lift your leg for 10 seconds. Do it 10 times on each side (3/minute).

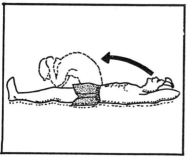

Sit-ups. Touch your elbows to your knees (5/minute).

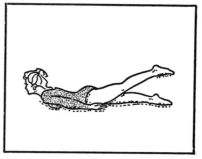

Lie face down and lift each leg 10 times (4/minute).

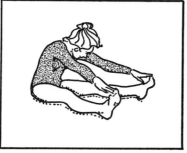

Sit up with your legs apart and bend forward to touch your toes 10 times (5/minute).

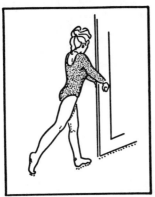

Hold on to the door knobs and swing your entire leg and thigh back and forth as far as you can. Repeat with the other lower extremity.

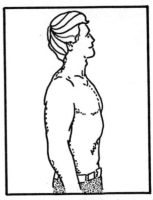

Hold in your abdominal muscles. Do it often.

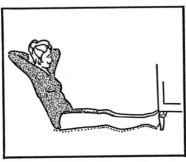

Lie down on the floor and wedge your feet under a piece of furniture. Place your hands behind your head and sit up and down.

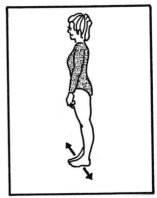

Stand with your feet together, keeping them flat against the floor, and try to pull them apart. Feel the strain against your outer thigh muscles.

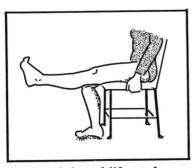

Sit in a chair and lift one leg out straight. This will tighten the anterior thigh muscles.

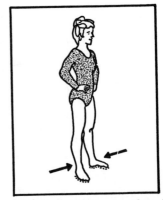

Stand with your legs apart keeping your feet flat on the floor and try to pull your legs together. Feel the strain on your inner thigh muscles.

Isometrics for Better Health

15 min. = 50 Pleasure Credits
Do each isometric for a count of ten.

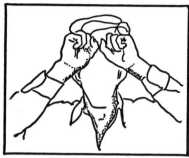

Place both fists against your forehead and hold it back as you try to
bend your head forward

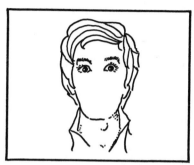

Open your eyes as wide as you can
and look momentarily in all directions without moving your head.

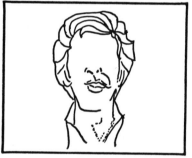

Alternately pull down each side of
your mouth.

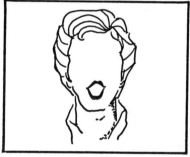

Open your mouth as wide as you
can.

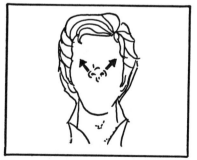

Flare-out your nostrils as wide as
you can.

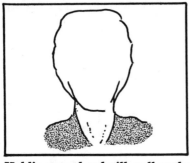

Holding your head still, pull up the muscles of the front of your neck and hold it.

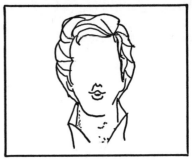

Purse your lips as if to whistle, using your facial muscles vigorously.

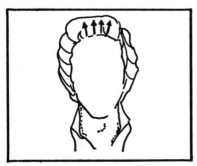

Pull back your scalp muscles so as to remove all the wrinkles of your forehead.

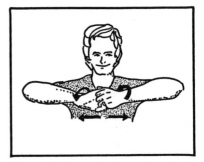

Clasp the fingers of your hands together and try to pull from side to side. Rotate one wrist against the other.

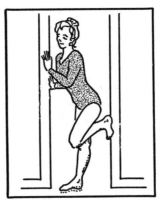

Find a place (i.e. corridor) where you can brace your body against a wall and push back with your leg against a wall behind you.

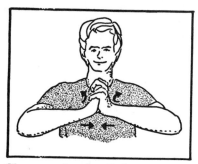

Clasp your hands together and press one hand against the other trying to move your arms from one side to another. Another variation is to try to bend one wrist back while resisting with the other.

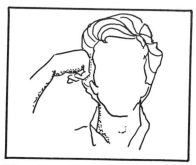

Place the palm of your hand against the side of your head and press as you try to bend your head to that side.

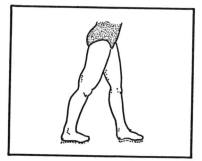

Stand with one leg behind the other and lean forward so you can feel the pull on the thigh muscle of the leg that is back. Repeat for the other leg.

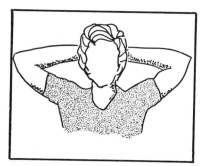

Clasp your hands behind your head and pull forward as you try to bend your head back.

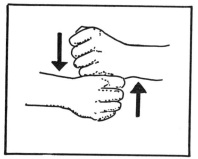

Place the fist of one hand on top of the other and press down.

Scene 4
Pleasure—Improving Your Expertise

Awareness is the expertise of living.

Pleasure is all around us . . . the problem is, we are not aware of it. The reason that it is absolutely necessary to write down the foods that you eat before you eat them, and put the Pleasure Units next to them, is that it makes you aware of what you are doing. It becomes the greatest safeguard of success and *permanent* weight loss. Because the "Pleasure Principle" is more than just a way of losing weight, your awareness must be extended throughout all aspects of your life. Pleasure must be obtained for the moment, but it can also be enjoyed in anticipation and in reflection. Awareness is focusing sharp and total attention on the "now." Usually our awareness is clouded by anxiety, depression, worry, concern, and all of the negative feelings we have talked about. In addition to the techniques described in Act II, Scene 3—The Only Way to Go, I have some specific suggestions to make in reference to the pleasure of eating.

SIX SENSES OF SATISFACTION

I have given lectures on sex education for many years in attempting to help people achieve the utmost satisfaction from sex. The word "sex," by the way, means pleasure; an approach which applies to all of our lives, including eating. Remember, "Achieve the Utmost Pleasure in Everything You Do, by Using Your Six Senses." To most people, the sense of *Taste* is the only sensation associated with eating. In reality, it is only one of six kinds of sensations that you can experience. The varieties are almost infinite. If you add to this all the variations of the other senses, the pleasure possibilities are incredible.

The *Smell* of food is often delightful and if you have ever tried to

194

eat when you had a cold you know how difficult it is to taste when you cannot smell. Gourmets describe the combination of taste and smell as the bouquet of food and drink. Think of how you can almost taste the food before you eat it just from the smell.

The *Touch* or texture of the food in your mouth can be a unique source of sensation. Think of the different feelings in your mouth when you bite a cold fresh apple, feel the crunch of crisp lettuce, or the velvety smoothness of ice cream. What marvelous pleasure and comfort you get from a hot cup of soup on a cold day or an ice cold drink on a hot day. No two foods are alike.

The *Sight* of food often stimulates the desire to eat. It can also satisfy that same desire. Many times when I have eaten out and used up my Pleasure Units for the day, I have had the waiter bring over the dessert cart so I could just look at the display. I am usually comfortable with what I have eaten, the amount has been adequate. I don't want to gain weight, so I'll just look at all the delicious cakes, pies and puddings and maybe say to myself, "Next time I think I'll have that cheesecake." I've had the pleasure of selecting, the pleasure of feeling comfortable, the pleasure of not exceeding my units for the day, the pleasure of knowing I can have it whenever I want it.

Food has a *Sound,* in fact, it has many sounds. There is a sound when you prepare it, a sound when you serve it, and a sound when you eat it. I am not referring to noises, I mean the pleasant sounds of living, such as the tinkle of glasses, the sounds of plates, the sizzling of bacon, the pouring of liquids, and the delightful crunch that you hear in your head as you munch on a raw carrot.

What is the sixth sense? It is the sense of *Feelings.* Food evokes feelings. There are foods that you love, foods that you hate, foods that make you feel silly, feel alert, or even feel passionate. There are foods that remind you of things, times, and places, both good and bad.

TIPS AND TECHNIQUES

In order to fully utilize all of your senses, there must be no dis-.ractions. This is where most of us get into trouble. How many times have you been out with friends, having a wonderful evening, and you were served your favorite dish. The chances are you took one bite, tasted it carefully and said, "This is about the best I have ever eaten." Then you probably resumed your conversation. At that moment, ninety percent of your attention was on your conversation and only ten percent was on what you were eating. You became absorbed in conversation and gobbled down your food; when finished, you felt full, but were left unsatisfied. When dessert time came, you were still seeking taste satisfaction, and stuffed yourself even more; but you were still not satisfied. What's the moral of the story? Don't talk when you eat. It is also a good idea not to listen when you eat. It is difficult for most human beings to do two things well at the same time. It is impossibe to give full concentration to either one of them. If you truly want to enjoy your food, then give it your complete attention. If you used all of your senses to enjoy your food, you could get five times the amount of pleasure while eating only half of the amount of food

There is another technique which will improve the ratio of enjoyment to the amount of food. Taste is experienced only in your mouth, and only as long as the food is in your mouth can the marvelous sensation of taste be appreciated. Foods and liquids must come in contact with the tastebuds of your tongue in order for the wonderful messages of pleasure to reach your brain. If you take a large bite, then much of what you are eating will not touch the tastebuds. The foods will be swallowed without giving you any pleasure. If, however, you take a small bite, roll it over your tongue, chew it *slowly*, concentrate on it, even have an orgasm with each bite, then you experience the maximum that food can offer in taste. If you take a bite of food that is half the size of the bite that you usually take, keep every bit of it in contact with your tastebuds for as long as possible, you can get ten times the amount of pleasure from half the amount of food. If you take large bites or eat quickly, then at least half the food you are eating is swallowed untasted.

You might explain these techniques to your friends the next time you have dinner. Tell them that you have discovered a new way of enjoying fattening food and keeping your weight down at the same time. Ask them to join you in an experiment. Suggest that when each course arrives, that everyone take small bites and concentrate on the flavor of the food in their mouth. Tell them to extract every bit of flavor from each bite. Explain that good conversation, like good food, demands your undivided attention. If you converse while you eat, you won't be able to enjoy your food. It is a terrible conflict to have to choose between good food and good conversation, so why do it? Why not separate the two so that they can both be enjoyed to the fullest? Your friends most likely will find this all amusing at first, but having tried it, I am sure they will agree with you.

A helpful technique in slowing down the pace of eating is to put down your utensils between each bite. The extra movement will help you burn up more energy and will serve to distract you less from the food that is in your mouth.

As you've learned to eat less and enjoy food more, you can also save a great deal of money. One technique that my wife and I have used while dining out is to order one appetizer each, but only one main dish and one dessert, which we share. You can adopt many variations of this technique by leaving out appetizers, ordering a main dish each and so on. You can leave out any of the courses, including the main dish and enjoy an appetizer, soup, salad, and dessert. How many times in the past have you wished you hadn't ordered a main dish by the time it came to the table? If you are going out for an evening of dining and conversation, why not order your appetizer, soup, and salad, and wait before you order a main dish? That way, you eat what you really want. I have always felt that far too much food is wasted in this country because of the excessive size of portions served by so many restaurants. Put an end to the uncomfortable, bloating sensations and the "I did it again" feeling that has plagued you so often in the past.

Think about your own energy requirements. Try to eat at least an hour before you are going to be burning up most of your energy input. It is not necessary, but it might help. Don't make life more difficult for yourself by placing excessive food on the table. Don't entice yourself into breaking your quest for pleasure. IF YOU WRITE IT DOWN BEFORE YOU EAT IT, WITH THE PLEASURE UNITS NEXT TO IT, YOU WON'T HAVE TO WORRY ABOUT OVERDOING IT ANYWAY.

Keep the Pleasure Unit List in your wallet or purse at all times. Keep it where you will always have it with you. If you should forget it, then guess at the value of the foods. Test yourself to see how well you have learned the foods you love. I have suggested to patients that they check off the foods that they usually eat on the Pleasure Unit List and then ask them to copy those into a small address book. They then have their own personal list that applies only to them. Ask those individuals who are usually with you at the time that you eat your meals to remind you to WRITE IT DOWN BEFORE YOU EAT IT. This is a pact that you have made, the single most important pact, if you want to lose weight. DO NOT BREAK IT! If you can't be bothered, then maybe you don't really want to lose weight. Type up the following pledge and tape it on your bathroom mirror. Read it every morning when you start your day.

Today I will find pleasure in every moment of life. I will eat whatever I want to eat, I swear I will write it down before I eat it. Living is a series of choices. I choose to be slender, I choose to be healthy, I choose a life of pleasure.

Scene 5
Pleasure Aids—A Helping Hand—
If You Still Need It!

LIVING THE PLEASURE PRINCIPLE

When you have accepted the concept that you can only live for today, and perhaps plan for tomorrow, then the depressing thought of the long haul no longer exists. The object is to live today, giving yourself pleasure from everything that you do, living a healthy, enjoyable life, and improving what you can so that this day is completely fulfilled and well-lived. Having lived a fulfilling day means that it has not been wasted, but has been lived to the hilt with total awareness of yourself and the world around you. By concentrating on living each moment and gaining pleasure from everything that you do, you leave little or no time to spend thinking about the disappointments of yesterday, which has no benefit. There is no worry about the possible consequences of tomorrow, which is likewise totally fruitless. If this day has brought you something unpleasant, disappointing, or depressing, you will have minimized it by the active search for pleasure and fulfillment. Whatever mistakes or failures occur in this day can be thought of as an education in life, a learning process and a means by which pleasure can be achieved the next time. If your mistakes or failures occurred during the search for pleasure, the search itself should have been pleasant and enjoyable, and the mistakes or failures become secondary. If you live only for the future, then all the effort you expend could be totally wasted. No one has tomorrow and tomorrow may not come. We only have today. You may plan for the future, and even enjoy that planning, but you cannot enjoy tomorrow until it comes; you can only enjoy today.

Anything that will help you safely lose weight is certainly worth trying. However, anything that you may try *must be in addition to the*

Pleasure Principle, and not instead of it. I say this not because other methods are ineffective, however they only work for roughly two out of every one hundred people. I've mentioned this fact numerous times throughout the book because I want you to know the odds will be fifty to one *against* your success in keeping the weight off for two years. You, your friends, neighbors, and others have proven that none of the existing methods of dieting will answer long-range needs, however, there are legitimate aids if you still need help in living the "Pleasure Principle will give you a brief rundown on the various techniques and methods that are available today. They are all safe, and all can be incorporated during either the period you are losing weight, or while you are maintaining it. If it turns you on . . . try it!

HYPNOSIS

For the past eighteen years, I have on occasion used hypnosis in my practice. I must admit however, that I frequently use informal techniques. A hypnotic trance takes many forms. It can occur without the subject knowing that he has been hypnotized, or it can be done in a very formal way, by such methods you are used to seeing on television or in a theater. Put simply, hypnosis represents the freeing of the subconscious mind from conscious control. A form of trance is common to all of us. A daydream represents a trance. It is a moment of inner preoccupation, when conscious control is lifted. It would appear that our conscious mind and its learned limitations keeps us from using the subconscious wish and drive for desired accomplishments. The success of hypnosis depends upon the needs and wants of the subject. For example, you may want to lose weight, but that does not mean that you want to give up the foods that you love. It is for this reason that most other methods have ultimately failed. The desire to lose weight for these individuals was only temporarily stronger than the desire to eat the foods they enjoyed. Once a reasonable amount of weight was lost, the desire to enjoy food again took over. Why create a conflict when none should exist? Keep this in mind if you go to a hypnotist for help. Be honest with him and tell him that you want to lose weight, but you don't want to give up eating good foods. Explain to him the "Pleasure Principle." Tell him that it is within this framework that you want to lose weight.

I don't think any hypnotist can claim that his clients lost weight permanently through negative suggestion. Negative suggestion is the technique used in which the hypnotist tells the patient that they will not have a desire for fattening foods. He may describe the foods under hypnosis as being unhealthy, distasteful, and nauseating. Some hypnotherapists even describe to their patients food covered with bugs and ants. These techniques may be successful, but only for a very short period of time. I would suggest that you ask your hypnotherapist to reinforce the basic rules that you must follow to achieve success in the "Pleasure Principle." He could constructively use the technique of reinforcing the Pleasure Unit limits when eating the foods you love. He could help you deal with the typical circumstances in your life that encourage you to eat as an inappropriate response. With hypnosis, he could sharpen your awareness of your unhealthy conditioning and help you lessen the frequency and intensity with which they occur. He could reinforce and encourage the accumulation of Pleasure Unit credits by encouraging pleasureful activities.

Hypnosis has come a long way from the "magical commands" that are supposed to rule your life. It has found its home in the field of psychology and medicine where it is becoming a highly effective tool in dealing with behavioral problems.

If you are afraid of hypnosis, your fear is probably based on a misconception. I know a few facts that will allay your fears. First off, you cannot be hypnotized unless you *want* to be hypnotized. Secondly, you will not accept a suggestion, unless you *want* to accept that suggestion, and it is reasonable and pleasing to you. (If you have watched a stage hypnotist and seen his subjects perform silly or funny acts on stage, it is only because they are willing and find it pleasant.) The third fact is that everyone can be hypnotized, but the experience is different for each individual; some people don't even realize that they have been hypnotized. (Under hypnosis the subject can still see, feel, speak, and think for himself.) Finally, hypnosis cannot hurt you.

I have prepared a hypnotic suggestion (see below). I would like you to read the following paragraph, and if you are willing to accept the suggestions made in that paragraph, then proceed with the instructions that follow

---

I will seek pleasure in every moment of life. It will be real pleasure. I will live my life only doing things that are in my best interest. I will write down everything I eat, before I eat it, with the pleasure units next to it. I am. I live my own life. I am successful.

In the evening, preferably just before bedtime, make yourself comfortable in a soft armchair. Place your feet flat on the floor. Place this book open to the next page on your lap and bend your forearms at the elbow so that your index fingers (your pointing fingers) point towards the ceiling. Comfortably bend your head forward so that your temples are resting on your index fingers. Look at a spot on the floor. Keep looking at it until your eyes feel tired and want to close. Let them close. When they are closed, take three deep breaths slowly. As you exhale each breath, let your body relax. With each breath, your body will relax more than the breath before. When your body feels totally relaxed, open your eyes and read the passage on page 200. You will feel as if the words and their meanings are entering your brain. You want them to and they will. When you reach the last word in the sentence, "successful," you will focus your eyes on that word and they will get tired and close. When they close, you will again take three deep breaths. With each breath you will feel completely refreshed, relaxed, and wonderful. If you wish at this time to go to sleep, you will have a wonderful, relaxed sleep. If you wish to do anything else, you will be able to do so with great ease and comfort. See yourself slender and trim, then open your eyes. You may repeat this process whenever you want to. It will strongly reinforce your conviction and your ability to carry out the Pleasure Principle.

DIET CLUBS

There must be a thousand diet clubs throughout the country. Most of them are based upon sound principles of nutrition. They all seem to have a reasonable degree of success with reference to losing weight. Their success in keeping the weight off is another matter entirely. I have yet to see statistics published by any of these clubs indicating their percentage of success in keeping weight off more than two years. Nevertheless, I believe that the "group therapy" offered by these clubs may provide some of my readers with the extra help needed to follow the "Pleasure Principle." None of these clubs offer the public what the public wants, and that is the opportunity to enjoy foods of one's own choosing while dieting and for the rest of one's life. It is for this reason I strongly suggest that you follow the Pleasure Principle and use the clubs as a means of maintaining incentive and developing the awareness I have referred to in this book.

PSYCHOTHERAPY

Most of us had spent at least twelve years in school. During this period of time we have developed our minds in the skills of reading, writing, mathematics, history, geography, etc. Unfortunately, not one moment has been spent on our feelings, on understanding ourselves, and in learning to cope with the problems of life. The aim of psychotherapy is to help you live your life to the best of your ability in a comfortable and healthy way. It is not a process in which you give your life's history and confess all your sins. It is an opportunity to express your feelings honestly and openly, without fear or condemnation. It is a method by which you achieve insight, establish awareness, and institute control. At one time, psychotherapy was a luxury to be enjoyed only by the wealthy. Today, it is available to virtually everyone. Your local medical society and your mental health association will be happy to assist you in obtaining help. There is no shame in going for help. Denying yourself that help *would* be a shame.

YOUR FAMILY DOCTOR

Personal medical care and the right to have a physician of your own choosing represents one of the great freedoms of our society. It gives you the opportunity to establish a sacred, confidential relationship with a physician that will fill your needs. Your family physician should be a trusted confidant, a learned and knowledgeable friend who will help you solve your health problems. He should be a source of guidance and comfort. His demands should be reasonable and realistic. Your demands should be the same. The Academy of Family Physicians was established to elevate and maintain the standards of excellence in family medicine. It was the first society to require continuing education. It constantly seeks to improve the knowledge and technical ability of its members. There are limitations, however, and it is in the freedom of choice of a physician that those limitations can be overcome. I speak primarily of those qualities of compassion, interest, and understanding which no one can legislate or teach. The feelings of trust, comfort, and confidence can be your only guideline, once you have established your physician's qualifications. Discuss the "Pleasure Principle" with him. Let him be a source of knowledge, guidance, and encouragement. Make it a rule to see him every two weeks. Show him your list and the count of Pleasure Units. Show him the essential rules; discuss them with him. Let him help you with any difficulties you may be having. By doing this, the trusting relationship that you and I hopefully established throughout this book will be continued through your personal physician. He will help you make minor adjustments to balance your eating patterns. These adjustments will ensure good healh and allow you to continue eating the foods you love. Your doctor's help and encouragement are important while you are losing weight, but it is often more important to talk with him *after* you have lost the weight. See him periodically, even if just to discuss how you are getting along. The bond between you should be a very special human relationship.

FAMILY AND FRIENDS

I am going to assume that your family is on your side and your friends are really your friends. If neither is true, you had best stay away from them. If you feel they are on your side, then it makes a lot of sense to sit down and discuss with them what you are going to accomplish. Try to ward off the obvious problems that usually arise by educating them "in front." Explain to them that though they mean well, they would only be hurting you if they encourage you to engage in deceptive pleasure. Tell them that you need all the help they can give you. You might explain that eating a "little bit more" is like being "a little bit pregnant." If a situation arises in which they try and encourage you to eat more than what you want, thank them, but be firm in your refusal. If they pressure you, thank them again, but tell them that you would appreciate it if they would not insist, because you *know* that they want to help, rather than hurt, you. If they persist after that, you may have to seriously question the motives of that individual, or their ability to cope with the positive changes in your life. *Calmly* inquire as to why they persist. Explain to them that you are comfortable and satisfied, and that if you eat more, you would feel uncomfortable and unhappy. Tell your friends how you feel, and no matter what they say, your feelings will not change. If you do weaken and give in, at least write the food down before you eat it. Although the reward for losing weight is the loss of weight itself, it is certainly meaningful when someone important in your life recognizes your accomplishment. It is more important to encourage you by praising your progress than by condemning your failures. Tell them this! The help from others however, should provide only encouragement; the motivation must come from within.

BEHAVIOR MODIFICATION

Behavioral modification therapy is an attempt at utilizing the disciplines of psychology, education and medicine in the understanding and treatment of unhealthy or destructive human behavior. The object of the behavioral patterns are acquired, performed, and changed. Their research and experimentation is carried out under strict scientific guidelines and research criteria. The behavioral scientist looks upon human behavior as being basically learned. They also believe that changes in behavior can be accomplished through the learning process and by manipulating the environment. In treating obesity, three basic approaches have been used. The first technique involves the use of aversion procedures. Favorite preferred foods are masked with repulsive or repugnant mental images, feelings, or odors. The second technique involves reinforcement of a favorable behavior with reward and unfavorable behavior with punishment. The reward usually involves words and gestures of approval or prizes in the form of money and valuables. Punishment is often in the form of condemnation, either from the individual therapist or from a group. In some instances, a type of physical punishment in the form of electric shock has been employed. The third technique involves the understanding and manipulating of the circumstances surrounding behavior. Several methods have been utilized in this category, and include the avoidance of stimulating situations, self-control and reinforcement, self-imposed deprivation, punishment, and monitoring and charting a behavior pattern.

Behavioral research has uncovered some fascinating data. Overweight subjects differed from their normal weight counterparts in many ways. They were more likely to eat according to a time schedule, they usually ate more quickly and in larger amounts, but less frequently. The amount of food that they ate was often determined by the amount of food available. It appeared that the obese were more influenced by environmental factors rather than by internal, emotional factors. Changing the environment therefore, involves changing a person's whole lifestyle. This would involve changing the food list, the food market, the route to and from the food market, the avoidance of food odors, and the sealing of food in opaque packages without pictures, as well as the time, place, and manner in which you eat and so on.

Maintaining weight loss appears to be as great a problem with the behavioral therapist as it is with all other forms of diet therapy. When the treatment ends, the dieting ends. The old habits reappear along with the weight. The Pleasure Principle offers an intelligent, simple way of utilizing the best of behavioral therapy, and creates a highly practical method of application so that weight loss and maintenance can be achieved permanently. Some of the techniques utilized in behavioral modification therapy are very sound and constructive. The monitoring of daily food intake, discussions of problems, and the education in nutrition and physical activity are all supportive and positive in effect. Other techniques involving food, special plates, methods, and times of eating, the dos and don'ts of special shopping lists, non-see-through containers hanging around the kitchen, etc., becomes a cumbersome, confusing, and discouraging approach.

POTPOURRI

In the past decade various techniques have been developed and have come into vogue, which might prove to be of great help in establishing the "Pleasure Principle" as a way of life. Books are available on each of these techniques should you be interested. I will simply list them and give you a brief description of what is involved. Depending upon your own personality and needs, one or more of these techniques may hold a definite attraction for you.

Consciousness-Raising Groups

These groups have been founded to counteract the guilt-confession concept of many diet clubs. Instead of saying that "fat is bad" or "you are unacceptable when fat," the consciousness-raising groups work towards raising self-esteem and eliminating self-punishment. They stress the fact that a person is worthwhile regardless of how much they weigh. They point out that being fat is to a great extent, a matter of choice. They concentrate on understanding, choices, consequences, and goals. They attempt to break the vicious cycle of being fat: social rejection — low self-esteem — self-punishment — depression — overeating — gaining weight and so on.

Overeaters Anonymous

I single out this particular club because they resemble the approach used by Alcoholics Anonymous and incorporate a strong religious flavor in their techniques. For those of you that are religiously inclined, this may prove to be of special interest.

Biofeedback

The term biofeedback was originally coined by researchers in the field of rehabilitation medicine. It originally utilized electronic equipment to help patients become aware of internal physiological events. These patients were taught to manipulate involuntary functions of the body. Biofeedback techniques were adopted by the so-called "mind control" groups in an effort to control behavior and feelings. It takes time and effort, and its value in weight reduction has not been established.

Assertiveness Training

This technique has been borrowed by psychologists and group therapists all over the country. The training involves a well-organized, systematic way of developing self-determination. It is based upon "Every Person's Bill of Rights." Everyone's rights are:

1. The right to be treated with respect.
2. The right to have and express your own feelings and opinions.

3. The right to be listened to and taken seriously.
4. The right to set your own priorities.
5. The right to say no without feeling guilty.
6. The right to ask for what you want.
7. The right to get what you paid for.
8. The right to ask for information from professionals.
9. The right to make mistakes.
10. The right to choose not to assert yourself.
11. The right to say "I don't know," "I don't care," and "I don't understand."
12. The right to offer no reasons or excuses for justifying your behavior.
13. The right to judge your own behavior, thoughts, and emotions.

The training then endeavors to help you with your problem areas, in dealing with life's situations, and in developing goals.

EST

EST is a potpourri marathon group of assertiveness training therapy, meditation, and brainwashing which was put together by an energetic, brilliant, former salesman. It has attracted over 150,000 followers. It uses a high pressure technique involving two weekend-long seminars, each day consisting of sixteen- to eighteen-hour sessions. It apparently has made 150,000 people feel as though they have greatly benefited from it. It has also caused at least seven known serious "psychotic breaks."

Transcendental Meditation (TM)

Transcendental Meditation is a highly commercialized organization that teaches a simple technique of meditation and gets you to pay for it by dressing it up in eastern mysticism. It is, however, a very effective technique of relaxing, relieving anxiety, and "recharging" the body. Simply described, it involves the use of a "mantra," a supposed personalized word which you repeat over and over again during the process of "meditation." This special work is somehow magically assigned to you by a trainer whose basic background is essentially no more than rote-memorization of the material he will repeat to you. My mantra was the meaningless word "har-eem." You have my permission to use it or any other meaningless word of your own choosing. The technique is simple and effective. Sit in a comfortable chair, place your feet on the floor and your hands in your lap. Relax and close your eyes. Repeat your meaningless word to yourself or out loud. Just keep repeating it. Your mind will have a tendency to drift and you will stop saying your mantra. As soon as you become aware that your mind has drifted and you have stopped saying the word, go back and repeat it again. If you keep doing this for about fifteen minutes, you will find it incredibly relaxing. You will very often find that it also gives you a new surge of energy. In dieting, this technique can be used to effectively combat the inappropriate messages of hunger that I mentioned earlier in the book.

DRUGS

Thyroid

Low-dose thyroid therapy is being reinvestigated. The T3 (Triidothyronine) factor in thyroid metabolism appears to be low during dieting. The thyroxine level from which T3 is made is not reduced during dieting. This would indicate that the conversion of thyroxine to T3 is not taking place at the usual rate. Some investigators feel that taking T3 might be helpful and even advisable during dieting. It is best to consult your doctor in this matter.

Appetite Depressants

Today, there are appetite depressant medications which do not stimulate the central nervous system. For some individuals they can be a safe, temporary help in getting started. I personally avoid them as much as possible in my practice; however, this again is a matter between you and your physician.

Bulk Tablets

Some studies have indicated that chewing the bulk, noncaloric tablets can significantly reduce the hunger intensity when you are losing weight. This can be particularly useful for individuals who are markedly obese and whose hunger seems uncontrollable. Because side effects are not serious (usually mild gastric distress, constipation, or nausea) it could prove to be a valuable aid.

Dilantin

Recently, the American Journal of Psychiatry reported on research done at the Stanford Student Health Service in Palo Alto, California. The investigation dealt with "binge eaters." The results were promising, but the long-term effect is unknown. "Binge eaters" impulsively devour huge amounts of food in a very short period of time. They appear to be incapable of controlling this behavior. If you truly fit into this category, your physician might look into this matter for you.

Spirulina

In 1981 considerable publicity was given to the appetite-suppressant effects of Spirulina. In view of the fact that no one, to my knowledge, has ever tested Spirulina, I have included the double-blind study which medical journals have for publication. Spirulina appears to have a definite appetite-suppressant effect in the majority of individuals who have tried it. Because it is a *food, a protein supplement,* Spirulina can be used in conjunction with the "Pleasure Principle Diet." It should be taken as follows: three tablets one hour before each meal. There are no known contraindications to taking Spirulina tablets.

Under the auspices of The Clinical Testing Center, Incorporated, a double-blind study was set up to verify the effectiveness of Spirulina in suppressing appetite. A field office for the company was set up in my office and an ad was placed in the Miami Herald seeking volunteers wishing to take part in a diet experiment. In view of the fact that Spirulina was classified by the FDA as a food, an investigatory number was not obtained. Spirulina has been used for centuries in both hemispheres, particularly Mexico, South America, and Africa as a food and a spice. It is currently sold throughout the United States in drugstores and health food stores as a nutritional supplement and is primarily a protein substance with a substantial vitamin and mineral content.

Interpretation of Results. Anorexigenic effect—based on the numerical values given to the answers on the questionnaire, the Spirulina group scored 3 to 1 over the placebo group. This represents a clear indication of an appetite-suppression effect from Spirulina. Of the nine patients in each group, six of the Spirulina group had a definite modification of hunger (no distinction was made between the words hunger or appetite—the distinction is one used mainly in the psychological professions and not by the lay public). In the placebo group only three of the nine indicated modification of hunger.

Although weight-loss is not necessarily a result of appetite suppression (it is determined more by total caloric intake or adherence to a diet which is a matter of discipline and choice), the weight loss for the Spirulina group was more than twice that of the placebo group.

Adherence to the diet was identical for both groups in terms of average days. Both groups stuck to the diet for nearly ten days (9.6 to 9.7) out of the fourteen day program.

Conclusion. Spirulina appears to have a significant effect on appetite suppression if taken in a dose of three tablets ½ hour before meals.

Starch Blockers

In 1981 an extract from navy beans was purported to have an enzyme that blocks the reception of starch (carbohydrates). Although many studies have been done on animals and many individuals have given testimony to the fact that they have been able to eat a reasonable amount of starch with their meals and still lose weight, many serious researchers are concerned with the possible effect that an enzyme-interfering substance might have on other enzymes of the body. The Federal Drug Administration, however, has cleared the starch blockers as a food supplement.

There you have it; take your choice! But remember, these are aids, not substitutes for the Pleasure Principle.

EPILOGUE
THE PLAY'S THE THING

So, there it is, leveled down to the nitty gritty; only three basic rules:

Eat the foods you love.
Lose weight comfortably.
Write it down before you eat it.

There is nothing dangerous to take; no rulings by the Department of Health and Human Services warning you of death and destruction, no lopsided diets that stress your system, and no cure-all regimen of chicken feed and dandelions guaranteed to not only make you lose weight, but also heal your boils and bunions.

I hope you can no longer be sold on the idea that someone can lose weight for you; I also hope you realize that you can lose weight on any diet, and that *your awareness* is the only guaranty of permanent weight-loss. But most of all, I hope that now, for the first time in your life, you are confident you can lose all the weight you want, and *keep* it off, using the "Pleasure Principle."

The "Pleasure Principle" is *your* way of eating *and* living!

The "Pleasure Principle" offers you the best of all possible worlds; A WORLD OF PLEASURE!

Don't just try it, DO it!

The "Pleasure Principle" works!

THIS WAS THE LAST PERFORMANCE, but it is not your last chance! There will be other books, other clubs, and other fads. There will be other promises and other claims. But what is going to change you? Don't turn your back on an opportunity to salvage your health. Don't wait until disease strikes. Next year may be too long to wait. The Pleasure Principle works!

It has always been hard for me to say good-bye. You have been with me for only a few short hours, while I have been preparing for those hours for almost a quarter of a century. An epilogue should be short, but I find it difficult to put my pen down. I hope you will pick up this book many times for reference. Most important, I deeply urge you to follow explicitly, with all your power and devotion, the few simple rules presented. They will insure success.

I know you've guessed by now, that Joe the Glut is really all of us. So, if you and I should ever meet, anywhere, anytime, and you say "Hi Joe," I'll smile. We understand each other and isn't it beautiful.

All the good maxims have been written.
It only remains to put them into practice.

Oh yes! . . . WRITE IT DOWN *BEFORE* YOU EAT IT . . . *AN* ∕
PUT THE PLEASURE UNITS NEXT TO IT!
If YOU WRITE IT DOWN AFTER YOU EAT OR AT THE END OF THE DAY . . . *IT WON'T WORK!* GOT IT? GREAT!

POCKET PLEASURE UNIT LIST

Directions: Cut out each section along the dotted lines and place each on top of the next in the order in which they appear, folding each section down the middle. Staple the entire pile of pages along the fold, creating a pocket reference of Pleasure Units for everyday use.

Food	Amount	Pleas. Units	Food	Amount	Pleas. Units
OIL & VINEGAR	1 T.	50	FRENCH FRIED POTATOES	1	15
ROQUEFORT CHEESE	1 T.	125	FRENCH TOAST	1 sl.	125
RUSSIAN	1 T.	50	FRUIT COCKTAIL	1 c.	100
DUCK	1/2	300	FRUIT PUNCH	1 gl.	200
WITH DRESSING	1/2	375	FRITTERS, FRUIT	1	200
DUMPLINGS, APPLE	1	275	CORN	1	100
E			FUDGE	1" sq.	100
ECLAIR	1	275	**G**		
EGGS	1	75	GEFILTE FISH	1	150
FRIED	1	100	GELATIN-JELLO		
EGGS CREOLE	2	175	ALL FLAVORS	1 c.	100
DEVILED	1	125	GINGER BREAD	SPP	175
EGG CREAM, CHOCOLATE	1 gl.	300	GRAPEFRUIT	1/2	50
EGG FOO YOUNG, CHICKEN	PP	250	GRAPES	1 c.	100
WITH PORK	PP	350	GREEN BEANS	1 c.	25
EGGNOG (BRANDY)	1 c.	300	GRAVIES, ALL	1 T.	50
EGGPLANT	1	50	GRIDDLE CAKES	PP	100
BAKED-ITALIAN	PP	350	GUAVAS	1	25
PARMIGIANA	PP	400	BUTTER	1 T.	50
EGG ROLL (CHINESE)	1	175	GUINEA HEN	1	175
ENCHILADAS	1	200	**H**		
ENGLISH MUFFIN	1	150	HADDOCK	PP	100
F			HAM	1 sl.	100
FIGS	1	25	DEVILED	1 T.	100
FIG BAR	1	50	HAMBURGER (ALL BEEF)	PP	200
FISH, SMOKED	1/2	150	FRIED	1 PP	225
FISH STICK	1	50	HASH, CORNED BEEF	1 c.	300
FISH, SWEET & SOUR	PP	200	HAZEL NUTS	1	10
FISH, WHITE, BROILED	PP	125	HERRING	bite size	25
FRIED	PP	225		1 strip	125
FLAVORINGS	1 t.	10	CREAMED	bite size	35
FLOUNDER	PP	100		1 strip	175
FRANKFURTER, ALL BEEF	1	125			
ROLLS	1	125			

Food	Amount	Pleas. Units	Food	Amount	Pleas. Units
COBBLER, APPLE	1	300	KALE	1 c.	50
COCOA	1 c.	125	KIDNEY BEANS	1 c.	225
WITH MILK	1 c.	250	KIDNEY/BEEF		
COCONUT			STEAK PIE	1 c.	250
MILK	1 c.	600	KIDNEY, BEEF	1 c.	200
WATER	1 c.	50	LAMB	1 c.	125
SHREDDED	1 c.	450	PIE	1 c.	225
CREAM	1 c.	800	KIPPERED HERRING	1/2	125
CODFISH	PP	100	KNOCKWURST	1	200
CODFISH BALLS	1	100	KREPLACH	1	75
COFFEE, BLACK	1 c.	0	KUMQUATS (FRESH)	1	15
COLA	1 gl.	100	**L**		
COLE SLAW	1 c.	25	LADY FINGERS	1	25
COMPOTE, APRICOT-APPLE	1 c.	100	LAMB, BARBECUED	PP	150
COOKIES			CHOP	1"	250
ANIMAL CRACKER	1	15	BREAST (STEWED)	1 c.	200
CHOCOLATE CHIP	1 med.	50	FRIED CHOP	1" thick	325
	1 lg.	75	LEMON	1	25
OREO	1 lg.	50	LETTUCE	1 head	50
ALL OTHERS	1	50	LIMA BEANS	1 c.	150
CORN, FRESH FROZEN	1 c.	150	LIVER, BEEF	PP	100
CORN FRITTERS	1	175	CHICKEN (CHOPPED)	1 scoop	200
CORN, CANNED	1 c.	150	PASTE	1 T.	50
CORN GRITS	1 c.	125	LIVERWURST	1 sl.	75
CORN ON THE COB	1	100	LOBSTER		
CORNED BEEF	PP	200	COCKTAIL	1 c.	175
CORNED BEEF HASH	1 c.	350	NEWBURG	1 c.	150
CRABAPPLES	1	50	TAIL, AFRICAN	1	100
CRAB, DEVILED	1	200	LOGANBERRIES	1 c.	100
CRABMEAT	1 c.	125	LONDON BROIL	PP	100
COCKTAIL	1 c.	200	**M**		
CRAB, SOFT SHELLED	1	100	MACARONI (BAKED)	1 c.	200
CRACKERS			WITH CHEESE	1 c.	450
CHEESE	1	15	MACAROONS	1	100
CHEESE SANDWICH	1	50			

Food	Amount	Pleas. Units	Food	Amount	Pleas. Units
HOMINY GRITS (COOKED)	1 c.	75	GRAHAM CRACKER	1	25
HONEY	1 T.	75	MATZOS	1 sheet	125
HONEYDEW MELON	1/4	75	MELBA TOAST	1 piece	15
HORSERADISH	1 T.	10	SODA CRACKER	1	15
HORS d'OEUVRES	sm.	25	THIN CRACKER	1	10
	lg.	50	TIDBITS, OYSTER	10	25
HOT CROSS BUNS	1	150	CRANBERRIES	1 c.	50
HOT DOG	1	125	SAUCE	1 T.	50
ROLL	1	125	**CREAM**		
I			HALF AND HALF	1 T.	25
ICE CREAM			NON-DAIRY	1 t.	10
ICE CREAM	1 scoop	150	WHIPPED, HEAVY	1 T.	50
ICE MILK	1 scoop	100	CREAM PUFF	1	175
FUDGSICLE	1 bar	100	CREAM SAUCE	1 T.	25
POPSICLE	1 bar	75	CROUTONS	1	5
ICECREAM BAR	1 bar	200	CRULLERS	1	150
CONE	1	175	CUCUMBERS	1	25
SANDWICH	1	175	CREPE SUZETTES	1	225
SUNDAE	1	400	**D**		
BANANA SPLIT	1	450	DANISH PASTRY	1	225
BISCUIT TORTONI	1	175	DATES	1	25
CAKE ROLL	1	175	DATE NUT BREAD	sl.	100
INDIAN NUTS	1 T.	25	DATES, STUFFED	1	50
ITALIAN BREAD	1/2" sl.	50	**DINNERS**		
			FROZEN	1	400
JAMS, JELLIES, PRESERVES,			WITH SAUCE	1	500
MARMALADE	1 T.	50	WITH DESSERT	1	500
JELLY APPLE	1	250	DIPS	T.	50
JELLY BEANS	1	15	DOUGHNUTS	1	150
JUICE, FRUIT	1 sm. gl.	100	FRENCH	1	200
VEGETABLE	1 gl.	75	JELLY	1	250
K			SUGARED	1	175
KAISER ROLL	1	125	DRESSINGS		
			FRENCH	1 T.	100

Food	Amount	Pleas. Units	Food	Amount	Pleas. Units
MALTED MILK	1 gl.	300	CHICKEN	1/2 sm. or PP	100
MANGO	1	100			
MAPLE SYRUP	1 T.	75	CHICKEN A LA KING	1 c.	750
MARMALADE	1 T.	50	CHICKEN CACCIATORE	PP	400
MARSHMALLOW TOPPING	1 T.	50	CHICKEN CHOP SUEY	1 c.	550
MARSHMALLOWS	1	25	CHICKEN CHOW MEIN	1 c.	250
MATZO	1 Round	75	CHICKEN FAT	1 t.	50
MATZO BALL	1	125	CHICKEN FRICASSEE	1 c.	225
MAYONNAISE	1 T.	100	CHICKEN (FRIED)	1/2	325
MEAT BALLS	1	100	CHICKEN LIVERS	1	50
WITH SPAGHETTI	1 c.	375	CHOPPED	1 T.	125
MEAT GRAVY	1 T.	25	CHICKEN POT PIE	1 c.	500
MEAT LOAF	1/2" sl.	225	CHICKEN SALAD	1 scoop	225
MEXICAN RICE	1 c.	225	CHICKEN PEAS	1 c.	150
MILK			CHILI CON CARNE	1 c.	500
ACIDOPHILUS	1 gl.	100	WITH BEANS	1 c.	350
BUTTERMILK	1 gl.	100	CHIPPED BEEF	1 c.	175
CONDENSED	1 T.	50	CHIPS, CRISPS AND		
DRY NON-FAT	1 gl.	75	SIMILAR SNACKS	1	15
EVAPORATED, CANNED	1 gl.	350	CHOCOLATE MILK	1 gl.	200
SKIM OR NON-FAT	1 gl.	100	CHOCOLATE PUDDING	1 c.	500
WHOLE	1 gl.	150	CHOP SUEY, PORK	1 c.	600
MILK SHAKE	1 gl.	350	CHOPPED STEAK	1/4 lb.	350
MILK TOAST	1 sl.	175	CHOW MEIN, PORK	1 c.	250
MINCE PIE	TPP	350	CHUCK STEAK (WITH BONE)	PP	100
MOLASSES	1 T.	50	CHUTNEY	1 t.	25
MOUSSE	1 c.	350	CINNAMON	1	0
MUFFINS, ALL	10	150	CINNAMON BUN	1	100
MUSHROOMS	1 c.	25	CINNAMON MUFFIN	1	100
MUSSELS	1 c.	100	CLAMS	1	10
MUSTARD	1 t.	10	CLAM BROTH	1 c.	50
			CLAM CHOWDER	1 bowl	275
N			CLAM JUICE	1 gl.	50
NAPOLEONS	1	300	CLAMS, STUFFED, DEVILED	1	20
NAVY BEANS	1 c.	200	CLAMS, FRIED	1	25
NECTARINE	1	50			

Food	Amount	Pleas. Units
FUDGE	1	100
GUMDROP	1	15
HARD CANDY (SMALL) LIFE SAVERS, SQUARES, ETC.		10
JELLY BEANS	1	10
KISSES, CHOC.	1	25
LOLLIPOP	1	100
MARSHMALLOW		25
MINTS		10
CHOC. COVERED	1	50
PEANUT BUTTER	SPP	100
CANTALOUPE	1/2	50
CAPON, ROASTED	1/2	225
CATSUP	1 T.	25
CAVIAR	1 T.	50
CEREALS, COLD	1 c.	125
COOKED	1 c.	150
CINAMMON TOAST	1 sl.	100
CELERY	1 stk.	5
COOKED	1 c.	25
CHEESE		
ALL	1 sl. or 1 oz.	100
CREAMED COTTAGE CHEESE	1 c.	250
CREAM CHEESE,	1 T.	50
WHIPPED	1 T.	25
AMERICAN, GRATED	1 T.	25
CHEESE SPREADS	1 T.	50
FARMER CHEESE	1 c.	400
POT CHEESE	1 c.	400
CHEESE BLINTZES	1	175
CHEESE SOUFFLE	1 c.	200
CHERRIES	1	5
CHESTNUTS (ROASTED)	1	5
CHEWING GUM	1 stick	5

Food	Amount	Pleas. Units
NOODLES, COOKED	1 c.	200
NOVA SCOTIA SALMON	1 sl.	200
NUTS, ALL	sm.	10
	1 lg.	25
	1 T.	25
NUTS, INDIAN		
LICHI		10
PINE	1 t.	25
O		
OILS, ALL	1 T.	125
ORANGE	1	75
SLICES	1 c.	100
OMELET	2 eggs,	150
	1 t. but.	185
ONIONS (BOILED)	1	50
CREAMED	1 c.	150
FRENCH FRIED	1	150
OVALTINE, WHOLE MILK	1 c.	225
OYSTER COCKTAIL	6	75
FRIED	1	50
RAW	1	10
P		
PANCAKES, WAFFLES & SIMILAR BREAKFAST FOODS		150
PANCAKES, GERMAN	1	225
PARFAIT	1	225
PARKERHOUSE ROLL	1	100
PARTY SNACKS	sm.	25
	lg.	50
PASTRY	each	300

Food	Amount	Pleas. Units
COCONUT	1 gl.	250
SHAKE	1 gl.	500
SKIM (LOW FAT)	1 gl.	100
OVALTINE	1 gl.	225
TEA	1 c.	0
BISCUITS	1	75
BLACKBERRIES (CANNED, SYRUP)	1 c.	200
BLACK-EYED PEAS (CANNED, DRAIN)	1 c.	200
BLACK WALNUTS	1	25
BLINTZES, CHEESE	1	175
FRUIT	1	100
BLUEBERRIES	1 c.	100
BLUEBERRY MUFFIN	1	150
BLUE CHEESE	1 T.	75
BORSCHT, BEET	1 c.	75
BOUILLABAISSE	Soup Plate	500
BRAINS	1 c.	200
BRAN MUFFIN	1	100
BRAZIL NUTS	1	25
BREAD	1 sl.	75
BREAD CRUMBS & STUFFING MIX	1 T.	25
BREADSTICKS	1	50
BROCCOLI	1 c.	50
BROWN BREAD (BOSTON)	5 PP	75
BRUSSELS SPROUTS	1 c.	75
BUTTER	1 pat	50
	1 T.	100
BUTTER COOKIES	1	25
BUTTER CRACKERS	1	25
BUTTER FROSTING (ANY FLAVOR)	1 T.	50
BUTTERNUTS	1	25
BUTTERSCOTCH SAUCE	1 T.	25

Food	Amount	Pleas. Units
SAUSAGE	1/6 of 12" pie, 1 sl.	250
PLUM	1	25
POPCORN	1 c.	50
PORK CHOP	1	225
PORK FRIED RICE	1 c.	225
PORK, KIDNEY	1 c.	150
PORK, LIVER	PP	150
ROAST	PP	200
SAUSAGE	1	75
SAUSAGE PATTY	1	175
SWEET & SOUR	1 c.	250
POSTUM (NO MILK)	1	50
POTATO, SWEET	1	200
MASHED	1 c.	175
HASH BROWN	1 c.	200
POTATO SALAD	1 c.	350
POTATO PANCAKE	1	175
POTATO, LYONNAISE	1 c.	400
FRENCH FRIED	1	15
BAKED	1	125
CHIPS	1	15
SLICED, FRIED	1 c.	500
AU GRATIN	1 c.	400
JULIENNE	1 c.	400
POT PIES (MEAT & CHICKEN)	1 whole	400
POT ROAST	PP	150
PRETZEL STICKS	1 thin	5
PRETZELS	1	20
PRUNES (COOKED)	1 sm.	25

Food	Amount	Pleas. Units	Food	Amount	Pleas. Units
TOASTEE	each	200	**C**		
PEACHES, CANNED	1	50	CANNED BEETS	1 c.	50
FRESH	1 med.	50	CABBAGE, BOILED	1 c.	50
SPICED	1	75	RAW	1 c.	50
PEANUT BRITTLE	SPP	75	STUFFED	1	150
PEANUT BUTTER	1 T.	100	CAKES (with nuts, add 50, with icing		
PEAR, ALLIGATOR	1	250	add 50)		
FRESH	1 med.	100	ANGEL FOOD	TPP	150
PEPPERS, GREEN (FRESH)	1	25	CHEESE	TPP	350
PERSIAN MELONS	1/8	75	CHOCOLATE	TPP	250
PERSIMMONS	1 med.	100	COCONUT	TPP	300
PETIT FOURS	1	100	COFFEE	SPP	100
PICKLES, DILL OR SOUR	1 sm.	15	CRUMB	SPP	100
OR SWEET	1 lg.	25	CUPCAKE	1	100
PIES			DEVIL'S FOOD	1/2" sl.	275
CHIFFON	TPP	275	ECLAIR	1	275
CREAM	TPP	400	HONEY	1/2" sl.	150
CUSTARD	TPP	200	JELLY ROLL	1/2" sl.	200
FRUIT	TPP	275	MARBLE	1/2" sl.	125
LEMON MERINGUE	Avg. piece	350	POUND	1/2" sl.	125
			SPONGE	1/2" sl.	125
POT-PIE, APPLE	1	400	STRAWBERRY SHORTCAKE	TPP	350
PUMPKIN	TPP	325	STRUEDEL	1	225
PINEAPPLE, CRUSHED	1 c.	150	UPSIDE DOWN	SPP	275
DICED	1 c.	100	WHIPPED CREAM	TPP	350
SLICED	1	25	ALL OTHER CAKES	TPP	200
PIZZA	1/6 of 12" pie,		WITH ICING ADD		50
	1 sl.	200	**CANDY**		
	snack size	25	ALL CHOCOLATE OR CHOC.		
			COVERED CANDY BARS	1	300
	1 sl.	225	BON BONS (CHOCOLATE		
ANCHOVIE			CREAMS, FRUITS,		
			NUTS, ETC.)	1	50
			CANDIED FRUIT	1	100
			CANDY APPLE	1	275
			CARAMEL	1	50

Food	Amount	Pleas. Units	Food	Amount	Pleas. Units
DRIED	4	100	**B**		
PRUNE WHIP	1 c.	100	BACON	1 strip	50
PUDDINGS	1 c.	400	BACON, CANADIAN	1 sl.	50
BREAD	1 c.	250	BAGEL	1	175
RICE	1 c.	350	BAKED ALASKA	1 c.	350
R			BAKED BEANS	1 c.	250
RADISHES	1	3	PORK OR MOLASSES	1 c.	350
RAISINS	1 T.	25	BANANA	1	100
RASPBERRIES	1 c.	100	SLICED	1 c.	125
RHUBARB (STEWED-NO SUGAR)	1 c.	50	BARBECUED BEEF	PP	150
RICE, BROWN	1 c.	150	BARBECUED CHICKEN	PP	150
CONVERTED, COOKED	1 c.	100	BARBECUE SAUCE	1 T.	50
CHINESE, FRIED	1 c.	200	BARLEY (COOKED)	1 c.	200
CUSTARD	1 c.	400	BEAN SPROUTS	1 c.	25
FRITTERS	1	50	BEEF, BOILED	PP	125
ROAST BEEF	PP	100	BEEF, CREAMED	1 c.	300
ROLLS	1	100	BEEF, CURRIED	1 c.	300
ONION	1	100	BEEF STROGANOFF	1 c.	300
PLAIN	1 lg.	100	BEEF STEAK & KIDNEY PIE	1 c.	300
S			BEEF STEW	1 c.	200
SALAD DRESSING	1 T.	75	BEET GREENS	1 c.	50
SALAMI	1/4" sl.	125	**BEVERAGES, COMMON**		
SALMON, BAKED	PP	250	CARBONATED (SODA)	1 gl.	100
CANNED	1 c.	300	CIDER	1 ql.	200
LOAF	1/2" sl.	225	COFFEE		
SAUCES	1 T.	25	EGGNOG	1 gl.	300
SAUERKRAUT	1 c.	50	FRUIT DRINKS	1 gl.	100
SAUSAGE	1 link	75	FRUIT JUICE	1 sm. gl.	100
SCALLOPS	1	25	(EXCEPT PRUNE)	1 sm. gl.	125
SEAFOOD, COCKTAIL	1 c.	150	TOMATO	1 sm. gl.	25
SHERBET, FRUIT	1 scoop	100	ICE CREAM SODA	1 gl.	275
			MILK	1 gl.	150
			(CHOCOLATE)	1 gl.	200
			COCOA	1 c.	175
			COCOMALT	gl.	275

Food	Amount	Pleas. Units
A		
A-1 SAUCE	1 t.	10
ABALONE	PP	100
ALCOHOLIC BEVERAGES		
ALE, BEER, MALT	1 gl.	100
COCKTAIL	4 oz.	150
GROG	1 c.	200
HIGHBALL	1 gl.	150
LIQUEUR & BRANDIES	1 oz.	100
WHISKEY	1½ oz.	100
WINE, CHAMPAGNE		
DRY	4 oz.	75
MEDIUM	4 oz.	125
SWEET	4 oz.	175
MIXED DRINKS WITH CREAM	1 gl.	225
ALMONDS	1	10
AMBROSIA	1 c.	150
ANCHOVY	1	10
ANCHOVY PASTE	1 T.	50
APPLE	1 sm.	75
APPLE, BAKED WITH SUGAR	1 sm.	200
APPLE, BROWN BETTY	1 c.	400
APPLE CIDER, HARD	1 c.	100
APPLE BUTTER	1 T.	50
APPLE SAUCE	1 c.	100
SWEETENED	1 c.	200
APRICOTS, FRESH	1	20
CANNED	1 c.	200
APRICOT BUTTER PRESERVES	1 T.	50
APRICOTS, DRIED	1	15
ARTICHOKE	1	75
ARTICHOKE HEARTS	1	50
ASPARAGUS	1	5
ASPARAGUS TIPS (CANNED)	1	5
AVOCADO	1 sm.	400

Food	Amount	Pleas. Units
SHISH KABOB	1 skewer	350
SHORTENING	1 T.	100
SHRIMP	1	15
FRIED	1	50
STUFFED	1	75
COCKTAIL	6	100
SIRLOIN STEAK	PP	100
TIPS, BEEF	PP	100
SMELTS (BROILED)	1	15
SNAPPER, RED	PP	100
SOUR CREAM	1 T.	50
SODA, ALL SOFT DRINKS	1 gl.	100
SOLE, FILET	PP	100
SOUPS		
BEAN	1 c.	150
BOULLION	1 cube	10
BROTH (CONSOMME)	1 c.	50
CHICKEN	1 c.	25
NOODLE	1 c.	50
GUMBO	1 c.	100
RICE	1 c.	50
CHOWDER	1 c.	75
THICK	1 c.	150
CREAM SOUPS	1 c.	150
PEA	1 c.	100
TOMATO	1 c.	75
VEGETABLE	1 c.	75
VICHYSSOISE	1 c.	100
SOY BEANS	1 c.	225
SPAGHETTI, PLAIN	1 c.	175
WITH SAUCE	1 c.	175
WITH 2 MEAT BALLS	c.	275

The Pleasure Unit List is presented in alphabetical order. In order to make it easy to use, many items in a particular category have been grouped together. For example, "ALCOHOLIC Beverages" contain all representative drinks such as beer, wine, cocktails, etc. "**Beverages, COMMON**", list almost all drinks such as soda, milk, malts, etc. CAKES, CANDY, COOKIES, CRACKERS, ICE CREAM, PIES, SOUPS and TOPPINGS have all been listed in a similar manner as general categories.

Food	Amount	Pleas. Units
PINEAPPLE	1 T.	50
FUDGE	1 T.	75
WHIPPED CREAM	1 T.	50
TROUT	PP	100
TUNA FISH (IN OIL)	1 c.	400
WATER PACKED	1 c.	250
TURKEY	PP	125
TURNOVERS, APPLE	1	250
V		
VEAL CUTLETS	PP	100
BREADED	PP	150
WITH CHEESE & TOMATO (PARM.)	PP	350
CHOP.	½" thick	150
MARSALA	PP	200
SCALLOPINA	PP	250
STEW	1 c.	250
VINEGAR	1 oz.	75
VEGETABLES		
ASPARAGUS	1 c.	25
LIMA BEANS	1 c.	200
BROCCOLI	1 c.	50
BRUSSEL SPROUTS	1 c.	50
CABBAGE	1 c.	25
CAULIFLOWER	1 c.	25
CARROTS	1 c.	50
EGGPLANT	1 c.	50
PEAS	1 c.	100
POTATOES	1 c.	175
SPINACH	1 c.	50
SQUASH	1 c.	100

ABBREVIATIONS

1 t.	=	1 teaspoon
1 T.	=	1 tablespoon
1 c.	=	1 tea cup
1 sm. gl.	=	1 juice glass
1 gl.	=	1 glass
1 sl.	=	1 slice (standard)
1 PP	=	1 Pleasure Portion
1 TPP	=	Triangular Pleasure Portion
1 SPP	=	Square Pleasure Portion

Remember: If you fry, add 50
If you bread, add 50

Food	Amount	Pleas. Units
WITH CLAM SAUCE	1 c.	225
SPARERIBS		50
SPINACH	1 c.	50
SQUASH, ACORN	1 c.	100
BUTTERNUT	1 c.	50
SUMMER	1 c.	50
SQUID	PP	100
STEAK, BEEF	PP	100
STEW, BEEF	1 c.	250
STRAWBERRIES, FROZEN	1 c.	25
FRESH	1	10
STRINGBEANS	1 c.	25
STRUDEL, APPLE	SPP	225
STURGEON	PP	150
SUGAR	1 t.	20
SUKIYAKI	1 c.	250
SWEET POTATOES	1	200
SWEET POTATO PIE	TPP	450
SWEET ROLLS	1	125
SWEETBREADS	1 c.	250
SYRUPS	1 T.	75
T		
TANGERINES	1	50
TOMATO (FRESH)	1 med.	25
JUICE	1 c.	50
ASPIC	1 c.	50
TONGUE, BEEF	PP or 1 sl.	150
TOPPINGS		
BUTTERSCOTCH	1 T.	50
CARAMEL	1 T.	50
CHOCOLATE	1 T.	75

Though a specific food may not be listed under a category, a typical example should be found. If you wish to find a ham sandwich, look up ham, bread, lettuce and mayonnaise and add them up. Various kinds of potatoes will be listed under "Potatoes, i.e., Potatoes, lyonnaise, Read through the list so you can become familiar with it and, therefore, quickly find the foods you want. If a particular dish is not listed, estimate the individual ingredients and add them up.

AND DEFINITIONS

=	$1/8$ oz.	
=	$1/2$ oz.	
=	6 oz.	
=	4 oz.	
=	8 oz.	
=	Packaged cheese, bread, salami, ham, etc.	
=	Portion the size of the palm of your hand; $1/4''$ thick.	
=	Measured by creating an imaginary triangle between the thumb and index finger.	
=	Measured by forming a right angle between the thumb and index finger. Base is the thumb length. Side is to the first joint of index finger.	

Food	Amount	Pleas. Units
W		
WAFFLE	1	225
WATER		0
WATERMELON	TPP	50
BALLS	1 c.	50
WAX BEANS	1 c.	25
WHIPPED CREAM	1 T	50
WHITEFISH, SMOKED	$1/2$	150
WIENER SCHNITZEL	PP	300
WON TON	1	100
WORCESTERSHIRE SAUCE	1 T.	25
YAMS	1	200
YOGURT, PLAIN	1 c.	175
Z		
ZABAGLIONE	1 c.	150
ZWEIBACK		35

PLEASURE PRINCIPLE
DIET

PLEASURE UNIT
LIST

COPYRIGHT 1977
ROBERT E. WILLNER, M.D.

Index